PRAISE FOR *MIKE & ME*

"*Mike & Me* is so beautifully written! The author illustrates how she and her husband chose to keep right on enjoying life after his Alzheimer's diagnosis. Hand in hand they took the leap of faith and embraced the journey together."
— **Laureen Rogers**, Professional Life Coach

"Rosalys Peel shows couples a path to a full and joyful life, despite one partner's Alzheimer's diagnosis. *Mike & Me* is the triumph of courage, grace and dignity over this discouraging disease."
— **Evelyn Williams**, *Blessings of Dementia*

"Here's proof that couples who are fighting the ravages of dementia can still have years of quality time together. As a behavioral neurologist who cares for many Alzheimer's couples, I highly recommend taking not just a page out of this book, but the whole thing!"
— **Glen R. Finney, M.D.**

"To know the road ahead, ask those coming back. Rosalys Peel provides every couple touched by Alzheimer's with vital information about what lies ahead. Her experiences with Mike show us how to live a full life together, even while facing a devastating illness."
— **Joni Powers, R.N., B.S.**, Integrative Medicine

"What a timely book! For thousands of couples who are now confronting Alzheimer's, *Mike & Me* shines welcome rays of hope into fearful and unfamiliar territory."
— **Doris Fleming**, Chaplain and Co-founder, Creative Expression Outlet

"Pragmatic and heartfelt, insightful and informative, *Mike & Me* reminds us that Alzheimer's, like life, is about hope, help and abiding love. It is a shared journey."
—**Bob Le Roy**, Exec. Director, Alzheimer's Assoc. Washington State Chapter

"Told with clear-eyed and loving honesty, *Mike & Me* describes a journey that no couple ever expects to take, but which comes to so many. Those just starting on the Alzheimer's journey as well as those well along will be profoundly supported and helped by this powerful and moving account."
— **Rev. Dennis Tierney**

"A treasured book of suggestions and guidance. *Mike & Me* provides vital new Insights into many aspects of Alzheimer's, including its impact on family, friends, and especially the patient's spouse."
— **Lawrence Murphy, M.D.**, Department of Neurology, Swedish Neurosciences

"The life skills, love and respect that Rosalys and Mike practiced over the course of their marriage are evident as they now decide how they will try to deal with Alzheimer's at home rather than in a care facility."
— **Caroline Stevens, R.N., M.S.W.**

"Mike Peel was my patient for more than a decade. This uplifting account makes me cry and smile as I remember how Mike and his adoring wife were able to confront Alzheimer's so effectively together. As I watch my own 93-year-old mother struggle with dementia, I am inspired to be a better caregiver, daughter and neurologist by Rosalys Peel and her wonderful book."
— **Lily Jung Henson, M.D.**

"*Mike & Me* is a tribute to how a loving couple and family found an inspiring new way to undertake the difficult Alzheimer's journey. Maintaining the dignity of the patient, providing a safe place as the disease progresses, pursuing needed resources—these critical issues are part of the wisdom in this lovingly written book."
— **Dr. Dianne Levisohn, M.D.**

"Thank you, Rosalys Peel, for opening your courageous loving heart to share your story and journey with the world. *Mike & Me* is an important book—an indispensable companion offering crucial insights for every couple coping with Alzheimer's—and doing so on your own terms with courage, grace, and endless love."
— **Michele Abrams**, Founder, In Concert for Cancer

"*Mike & Me* provides tangible ways to ease the challenges of Alzheimer's and live each day fully despite a life-limiting illness. It's an inspiring and profound example of how great joy and beauty can come with (and often through) hardship or suffering. I highly recommend it!"
— **Natalie Rodden, M.D.**, Hospice and Palliative Medicine Physician

"A courageous account that brought tears of joy to my eyes. Each chapter details how love and commitment really can prevail over this deadly disease."
— **Tom Gorman**, former US Davis Cup Coach

"Knowing we have options and choices when confronting Alzheimer's is empowering. Rosalys Peel offers a vivid and loving picture of one couple's decision to live with Alzheimer's in their own way. This book is sure to help many other couples."
— **Trudy James**, Chaplain, Producer of *Speaking of Dying* film

"*Mike & Me* is an immediate, practical and essential lifeline for any couple who decides to tackle Alzheimer's together at home. The author's insights on the legal and financial concerns that every Alzheimer's couple faces are worth the price of the book alone."
— **Jesse Robeson**, Attorney

MIKE & ME

AN INSPIRING GUIDE FOR COUPLES
WHO CHOOSE TO FACE ALZHEIMER'S
TOGETHER AT HOME

ROSALYS PEEL
WITH DAN ZADRA

An imprint of Zadra Creative, LLC
513½ Bank St.
Suite A
Wallace, Idaho 83873

For information about quantity discounts on bulk
purchases, contact Zadra Publishing, at 206.551.3618,
or Dan@ZadraCreative.com

Rosalys Peel is available for book signings, or selected Alzheimer's
speaking events at 206.551.3618

Cover and Interior Design by
Toby Cowan, Performance Design Group
Sebastopol, CA

Front cover photo by View Apart/Shutterstock
Back cover photo by Katie Brase

Edited by Luana Cowan

Library of Congress Control Number: 2017917783

ISBN # 978-0-692-04678-4

FIRST PAPERBACK EDITION
Printed in the United States of America

THIS BOOK
IS DEDICATED
TO YOU

Each year, thousands of American couples are given the disheartening news that a spouse or partner has been diagnosed with Alzheimer's. If you are one of these couples, this book is dedicated to you and your loving family and friends.

It's empowering for Alzheimer's couples to discover that there is more than one way to confront this disease together. In that respect, *Mike & Me* is not just a book, it's a "way."

When Mike was diagnosed with Alzheimer's we made a pact to stay in our own home and to find a way to continue living a full life together. We had no idea how our "stay-at-home" choice would turn out, but we did know we could always turn to one of many excellent Alzheimer's care facilities if it didn't. The lessons we learned are here for you. May they inspire and guide you and your loved one on the journey ahead.

I am grateful to the entire Alzheimer's community—the growing legion of researchers, doctors, nurses, counselors and caregivers who are creating better lives for those fighting this disheartening disease. It's a privilege to share the unique story in these pages, along with fresh information and guidance for Alzheimer's couples everywhere.

In loving memory of Mike Peel
May 23, 1935 to June 6, 2011

CONTENTS

PROLOGUE

~

DEAR READER:

If you and your loved one are
thinking about dealing with
Alzheimer's together at home, you've
picked up the right book.
Let's get started.

WHEN MY LOVING HUSBAND MICHAEL, to whom I was married for 45 years, was diagnosed with Alzheimer's, I started keeping a journal.

At first I was just trying to record new information and treatment advice from our doctor. But it turned out that journaling became a very empowering and comforting companion for me over the entire nine-and-a-half years that Mike and I dealt with his Alzheimer's.

My journal was a safe place where I could give words to my worries, concerns and fears. It's where I logged the frustrations and setbacks that Mike and I encountered, but also where I recorded and celebrated our many victories, large and small.

Over time, I became aware that our journey with Alzheimer's was different in certain ways from the experiences other couples were having. You see, Mike and I had decided that, despite Alzheimer's, we would go right on pursuing our hopes and dreams, and we would confront the disease together in our own home, one day at a time. I searched high and low for good information to help guide us on that journey, but I found very little.

That led to the birth of an idea: I decided to journal more instead of less, with the thought that someday I might leave a helpful road map of vital information and guidance for other Alzheimer's couples to follow. What this guidance would look like was an unknown at the time; perhaps it would be a little pamphlet with a few tips, or maybe a short story about our journey.

Later, I had a chance meeting with an experienced and caring writer who gave me this quote by author Toni Morrison: "If there's a book that you want to read, but it hasn't been written yet, then you must write it." The book you now hold in your hands is the result.

TAKE THIS BOOK WITH YOU ON YOUR JOURNEY

Today, whenever I tell people that I lost my husband Mike to Alzheimer's, I see the concern wash over their faces. Perhaps like you they have heard the usual horror stories associated with this disease, and they just assume that Mike and I must have had a devastating journey together. But I am always quick to tell them that it wasn't that way for Mike and me.

The truth is, Mike and I went a long way together—as far as the road would take us—and this book will show you how. He died in the end, but he died as we all want to die—with grace and dignity. And not before we experienced years of life and love together.

Mike and I completed our nearly 10-year Alzheimer's journey together, and now I have returned from the journey to tell you the simple but hopeful lessons that my husband and I learned along the way; and to share how our Alzheimer's experience was much different from the typical horror stories we have all heard.

Whether you are the one with the illness, or the one who is the partner providing the care, I now know that what Mike and I did and how we did it will help you on your journey too. The decision to manage Alzheimer's together in your own home, for either all or part of the journey, may not be the right choice for some, but I now know that it should be a viable consideration for all.

Your journey will no doubt be different from ours in certain ways and yet the same in others, for we are now all members of the same brave club. We have all had the same fears and worries: "Can we really do this, and how will we do it?"

I am here to tell you that you can. You've picked up the right book, so let's get started.

Rosalyn Peel

A GUIDE FOR THE ROAD AHEAD

*For Mike and me, our challenge (and
now yours) was to set out on the
Alzheimer's journey together—and
to keep hope alive.*

EVERY NOW AND THEN EVEN THE HEALTHIEST COUPLES
will stop for a moment and ask, "What if?" What if one of us has
a stroke? What if one of us has a heart attack? What if one of us is
diagnosed with cancer?

Mike and I asked ourselves those same questions through the
years but, perhaps like you, we never asked, "What if one of us gets
Alzheimer's? What then?"

Each year, thousands of American couples are blindsided by this
disheartening disease. I say "couples" because no husband or wife
ever makes the Alzheimer's journey on their own; their partner is
there too. The moment one partner is diagnosed, the other partner
joins the journey. This is not something someone does alone.

When my husband Mike was diagnosed back in 2002, the pre-
vailing opinion in the medical community at that time was that
most people with Alzheimer's will sooner or later have to leave their
home and go live in a care facility. Mike said to me, "I don't want to
leave you and our home." I said, "I think we can do this at home."
But, could we?

In part, *Mike & Me* is the story of my husband's incredible
spirit, courage and sense of humor in the face of a potentially lethal
disease. But the main focus in these pages is to chronicle our
mutual commitment to do all that we could to prevent this disease

from progressing—and to keep our marriage alive and our home life intact.

If you are a loving partner in an Alzheimer's relationship, I'm sure you already know why Mike and I decided to defy the odds and stay together as long as possible in our own home. This book has been written to share how we did it, and to help you learn how you might do it too.

WHAT TO EXPECT IN THE PAGES AHEAD

I have learned that every couple's Alzheimer's story is different. This disease has a way of taking unexpected twists and turns, not allowing us to know exactly which way it is headed next. Because each couple's path is different, you do not get to know exactly how your journey will go—nor did Mike and I get to know ours. But there are important signs and similarities to look for in all who are ill, and I will share those with you in the pages ahead.

About the only thing Mike and I knew for sure when we first started our journey was that someday there would be a cure for Alzheimer's. We hoped it would be in our time, but our time eventually ran out. Through the years, however, we succeeded beyond all expectations to keep the "we" in our relationship, and we were still "us" to the very end.

For you and your partner, there may still be a cure in the near future, and it may well be in time. No matter how or when that possibility works out, however, you can decide right now that you will take control as a couple and learn how to work through the challenges together as this disease progresses. I want to assure you that the powerful, loving "we" in your relationship can continue through thick and thin, and that it is possible to keep that "we" until the very end.

For Mike and me, our challenge (and now yours) was to keep hope alive as we moved forward with our lives. Never despair. Keep looking for the joys in every day—the subtle joys and gifts that others might miss—and keep looking forward to what tomorrow will bring for both of you. In that way the journey can continue with mutual love, meaning and dignity as you walk this difficult path together as partners in life.

"LET'S GET ON WITH IT"

Another thing I now know for certain: when faced with adversity, we humans really are incredibly resilient and resourceful, especially when we stick together. We all have unique gifts and strengths that we can draw on when we are challenged or afraid. Mike and I discovered our gifts along the way, and I promise that you will discover yours too.

Mike's gifts were many, partially because he had already experienced significant difficulties in his life. He had always survived and prevailed in the past, so he naturally decided he could do this with Alzheimer's too. He made up his mind in the beginning how he would manage the illness, and this approach worked for him and for me.

After the initial diagnosis, Mike experienced a period of disbelief and anger, but he then said, "Let's get on with it," and we did. Together, we made the most of each day until the very end, and that made all the difference.

The gifts I brought to our Alzheimer's journey were different and unexpected. Part of my background is in nursing, but that didn't really play a big part because I hadn't provided patient care for many years. Surprisingly, it was my experience as a parent educator and couples' relationship facilitator that eventually provided Mike and me with some of the missing tools we needed to deal effectively with Alzheimer's.

During the early stages of Mike's illness, I was helping to create the couples' relationship workshops at Swedish Medical Center in Seattle. These workshops are based on research by Dr. John Gottman, the best-selling author of *Seven Principles for Making Marriage*

Work. They are designed to help couples strengthen their relationship and develop an effective way to handle conflict, especially in times of stress or hardship.

It turned out that some of these same insights helped Mike and me preserve our long-standing relationship despite the stresses and hardships of Alzheimer's. I look forward to sharing these and similar insights with you and your partner in the pages ahead.

PART I

~

Discovering Mike
Has Alzheimer's

CHAPTER 1

WHAT'S WRONG WITH MIKE?

*A continuing pattern of foggy
thinking and forgetfulness eventually
led to a startling diagnosis.*

EACH YEAR APPROXIMATELY 450,000 PEOPLE are formally diagnosed with Alzheimer's in the U.S. alone, and the numbers are on the rise. More than ever before the discouraging images of Alzheimer's patients in decline are now featured in the media, leaving all of us saddened and on edge. If we forget where we left our keys, or can't remember someone's name, or don't recall why we walked into a room, we begin to worry, "What's wrong with me? Do I have Alzheimer's?"

For the majority of people, of course, those worries are empty balloons. But, for Mike and me, a continuing pattern of foggy thinking and forgetfulness on Mike's part eventually led to more serious concerns and, finally, to a startling diagnosis.

I want to share the timeline leading up to that diagnosis in this chapter so I can give you a useful snapshot of how our subsequent journey with Alzheimer's progressed. Again, while our journey will differ from yours in certain ways, my hope is that one aspect will be the same: Mike and I decided to travel the road together, with love and dignity from start to finish, and that mutual decision ultimately made all the difference in the quality of our remaining years.

HOW WE DISCOVERED MIKE HAD ALZHEIMER'S

Believe it or not, the initial concerns surfaced nearly four years before we received the formal diagnosis of Alzheimer's. I began to notice that Mike was having more than simple memory issues. I might have to say something three times before he "got it." Our friends and family chalked it up to plain old forgetfulness. More and more, however, Mike was not responding to what I said, and not following through with things he did hear. This was becoming a chronic problem for us. To make matters worse, he didn't understand what I was upset about, and I didn't understand why he didn't follow through on the things we talked about. (At this point, you are probably thinking that you, too, have Alzheimer's. But hold on—not so fast.)

For a while Mike tried to solve his "forgetfulness" problem by simply jotting things down in a little notebook to jog his memory. When that didn't work, we both finally acknowledged that we needed help figuring this out. We made an appointment with our nurse practitioner and told her about the difficulties we were having. She thought the culprit might be hearing loss or sleep apnea and scheduled the appropriate tests.

Mike's hearing tests took weeks to finalize, but it was finally confirmed that his hearing was fine. I was told that I just needed to talk to Mike up close, and he just needed to be more focused. Hmm.

From there, we turned to sleep apnea as the potential problem. Mike spent a night at the sleep study clinic and—sure enough—he did have sleep apnea. We were set up with a CPAP (sleep apnea machine) which he had to use at night. It was frustrating for Mike, but at least we were now hopeful that we had found the cause of his mental lapses. He simply had sleep apnea, and life would soon get back to normal with the magic CPAP machine. But it didn't.

For Christmas that year we surprised our young adult children, Kathleen and Patrick, with the gift of a January trip to Hawaii. Mike and I would go along to share the adventure of our kids' first trip to the islands. How could we not enjoy a trip to Hawaii in the middle of a gray northwest winter? It was going to be wonderful!

With enthusiasm, we practiced packing the CPAP machine (with mask, cords and plugs) into a backpack, and thought all the trip preparations were covered. Then, out of the blue, Mike announced that he didn't think he could go. He had a contract with a company that had given him some deadlines for work to be done and reports written. It seemed that Mike was having a problem completing the work to their satisfaction and had some reports sent back for him to properly redo.

Eventually, he decided that he could make the trip to Hawaii, but would have to bring his work along. Okay, I guessed that would have to be the way it would work. He assured me that his work would not interfere with our trip and, because I wanted him to come, I believed him.

A reality check came our first day in Hawaii. While the children and I went to the beach, Mike stayed in our family-friendly condo to work on his reports. Later, when I offered to proof his work, I saw immediately that his reports were disorganized and difficult to read. The next day, when our son Patrick offered to stay at the condo to help, he, too, discovered that Mike was having major problems with basic writing.

Patrick, who had been away for four months, told me privately that he now felt his dad was worse than the last time he had seen him. That was helpful information because I was apparently too close to the situation to recognize how things were deteriorating. Every day, now, I worried, "What's wrong with Mike?"

OUR CONCERNS INCREASE

After our Hawaii vacation we went back to our nurse practitioner for advice. This time we were referred to a neurologist. After multiple appointments, an MRI and other lab tests, the doctor gave us the results of Mike's neurological workup. Good news! The results were all negative; Mike apparently did not have a neurological problem. The neurologist said he didn't really know what was wrong with Mike, but it was not Alzheimer's. He prescribed conventional anti-depressants. Antidepressants? We were both relieved to hear Mike did not have Alzheimer's, but was it really depression?

After that doctor's appointment, we walked down the hill to the ferry in silence. When we stopped at a crosswalk, Mike turned to me and said, "Do you think I'm depressed?" I said no, and Mike never did take those antidepressants.

We returned to our nurse practitioner once again. This is probably sounding familiar to you because virtually every Alzheimer's couple I know or hear about has had a similar frustrating and meandering experience on the road to the final diagnosis.

In our case, our nurse practitioner convinced us to get a second opinion from a different neurologist, Dr. Lily Jung. After four years of wondering, "What's wrong with Mike?", it was Dr. Jung who finally sat down with us and said, "I'm pretty sure this is Alzheimer's." The emotional impact of her conclusion was both devastating and confusing. (More on that in the next chapter.)

It was confusing because we now had two different medical opinions—depression and Alzheimer's. And because we did not want to believe it was Alzheimer's, we went to the University of Washington Medical Center for yet another opinion. After a new string of tests, the doctors at the University told us that, while they still couldn't be absolutely sure, they, too, thought it was Alzheimer's.

Still no one-hundred-percent conclusive diagnostic test, but our hopes were now dwindling. At that point we returned to Dr. Jung, who would remain Mike's trusted doctor for years to come, providing the skill and loving care that is needed with this complicated illness. Dr. Jung decided to prescribe an Alzheimer's drug called Aricept. She said that if Mike responded positively to Aricept, it would be another key indicator that he did, in fact, have the disease.

In March, we had a follow-up visit with Dr. Jung, and she confirmed that the Aricept seemed to be working. Our daughter Kathleen reported that, with Aricept, her dad could now order lunch and knew what he wanted and how he wanted it. And I reported that Mike could now focus on what I was saying and that I didn't need to repeat my sentences three times.

Because Mike couldn't perform those tasks and others competently without Aricept, the results were conclusive. We now had to face our fears. What was wrong with Mike was Alzheimer's.

<hr />

INSIGHTS

- While searching for the final diagnosis, I learned many things along the way, including: Alzheimer's is just one of many forms of dementia, so it can be difficult to diagnosis.

- Because there are many forms of dementia, the doctor is on the hunt to pinpoint the real problem. Once the problem is officially diagnosed as Alzheimer's, only then is it possible to effectively start treating the illness.

- Your loved one's increasing inability to recall things is typically a key symptom or "clue" that he/she may be developing Alzheimer's. It turns out that the collective experiences of all family members can combine to provide a clearer picture of whether or not recall seems to be deteriorating. In our case, for example, our son Patrick (who had not seen his dad for a while) was able to help us assess that his dad's memory was definitely getting worse.

- A hearing problem is frequently one of the first complaints of Alzheimer's couples. So if you really feel there is a hearing problem, but the first hearing test is negative, then seek a second opinion. Don't be content with, "You just need to focus or listen better."

- As new research dollars pour in, things are changing for Alzheimer's patients. For example, we may soon be able to diagnosis the disease much sooner. Be sure you have a neurologist who stays current on the latest discoveries and improvements. Get on the Alzheimer's Alert list, and stay current yourself with what's in the news. For the most part, good news is on the way.

- Early diagnosis is becoming more frequent and accurate today. And, once diagnosed, people are being treated with more effective lifestyle choices and changes to slow progression of the disease.

- By all means you should feel comfortable getting a second or third opinion. Alzheimer's can be difficult to diagnose. Getting that second opinion can give you the same certainty—one way or another—that Mike and I needed to move forward with our lives.

- Finally, keep hope alive. As I write this, there are teams of researchers who are closing in on new treatments to slow or perhaps even stop the disease—and many believe they are almost there. So remain optimistic and forward looking. By all means, continue to pursue your dreams, stay healthy and active, enjoy each day and look forward to each tomorrow.

- Remember always that you are not alone on your journey. More and more our entire nation is coming together to find solutions to this disease and help those who are fighting.

CHAPTER 2

THE DAY WE GOT
THE DIAGNOSIS

---

*Alzheimer's! The word itself is big
and haunting. Hearing the formal
diagnosis that day triggered an
immediate mix of raw emotions, new
fears and uncertainties.*

THE DAY YOU OR YOUR PARTNER HEAR that you have Alzheimer's is like no day you have experienced before or will experience again. Shock and disbelief arrive first and then your hearing seems to short circuit, making it impossible to comprehend what the doctor says next.

Looking back, I remember Dr. Jung coming into the room and sitting down with Mike, Kathleen and me that day. Quietly but firmly she explained that, after reviewing the latest neurological tests, she thought Mike did in fact have Alzheimer's. She said a few other things after that, but I have no idea what they might have been. My mind was racing. I thought, "How can it possibly be Alzheimer's? Just a year ago we were assured it was *not* Alzheimer's!"

I remember Mike, Kathleen and I all fell into silence together. After sitting with us for a short time Dr. Jung said, "I'll be right back" and stepped out of the room. She was gone for quite a while and I now realize she was giving us time and space to absorb what we had just been told.

While the doctor was gone, we began to assure each other that this was not possible—that it must be a mistake. Maybe it was depression like the previous doctor had said. (At that point a diagnosis of depression was sounding like a blessing because we could fix depression—and we all knew there was no fix for Alzheimer's.)

By the time Dr. Jung returned we had formulated our thoughts and questions, especially, "How do you know it's Alzheimer's?" Dr. Jung replied that the way Mike had been responding to the assessment tests ruled out depression. Plus, the way we (his family) had been reporting the steady decline of his memory was consistent with Alzheimer's.

It's difficult to remember all the emotions that ran through my mind that day. What Mike and I felt and said is a blur, but I remember it helped to have our daughter there. We did not cry that day; those tears would come later. We left in disbelief and slight defiance, vowing we would get a second opinion to see if the diagnosis was correct.

It turned out that seeking that second opinion at the University of Washington Medical Center a few weeks later helped get our feet on the ground and prepared us for the new journey ahead. By then, we had slowly settled into the stark reality that the Alzheimer's diagnosis was accurate. When the Medical Center assured us that this was the case, we finally accepted the verdict as bravely as possible—and then began to gather our strength to deal with this new reality.

INSIGHTS

- Some people fear diagnosis so much that they actually put off going to the doctor. They would rather not know if something is wrong.

- Try to see diagnosis as an alarm that has gone off in your home. Yes, the alarm is telling you that something dangerous has entered your world, and that's pretty scary. But at least now you have been alerted and can deal with it.

- Every journey begins with the first step. By seeking and securing a clear diagnosis, you and your loved one have already taken that all-important step.

CHAPTER 3

HOW LONG DO WE HAVE?

*Once Mike and I had accepted the
diagnosis as real, two big
questions arose.*

MIKE WAS DIAGNOSED BY DR. JUNG IN JANUARY, 2002 at
Seattle's Swedish Neurological Institute. This was nearly four years
after we first noticed something was wrong with Mike's cognition.

After we calmed to the diagnosis, the first obvious question was,
"How long do we have?" We were told at that time that people with
Alzheimer's typically live about nine years after diagnosis, and that
the last two years are usually spent in a 24-hour care facility. Learning that we probably still had a number of good years ahead of us
was somewhat reassuring. It was neither a long time, nor a short
time. But Mike and I both felt it was time enough to continue pursuing some of our dreams, to make plans for a meaningful future,
and to hold out hope for new medical advancements or even a cure
along the way.

Today the Alzheimer's Association gives a fairly large range in how
long someone might live with Alzheimer's. No two people are identi-
cal, so trust your doctor to give you some useful statistical estimates
for your personal circumstances. You'll find that having an estimated
time frame can help you gauge the best life choices, going forward.

But here's a word of caution: Don't buy in to strict time limits,
for they tend to become a self-fulfilling prophecy. The truth is, neither you nor your physician knows exactly how much time you and
your loved one have been allotted on this earth. Who knows how

well you might adapt to the disease and exceed expectations? Who can tell where medical research will be in a year, two years, or five years from now? So, pay attention to the latest guidelines and statistics, but do not consider them cast in stone.

WHEN WILL IT GET DIFFICULT?

The second question that arose right after diagnosis was, "When will life start getting difficult with this disease?" Life for us was not difficult when Mike first got the diagnosis. True, he often forgot things, or misplaced things, or couldn't recall what I told him, but we were still able to enjoy a somewhat normal life like most couples. So the pressing question for both of us now became, "How long will our life continue to remain somewhat normal—and when might it become more difficult?"

Most in the field of Alzheimer's describe the last two years as the most difficult and I would agree. But I would also say that the last eight to ten months of Mike's illness were the hardest.

And yet—and this is such an important realization—Mike and I were never more in love, or more tuned into each other than the last year of his illness. As you will see in upcoming chapters, those final months hold tender memories for me, and I know they were tender times for Mike too.

For now, just know that you, too, can make the Alzheimer's journey more positive than negative, and that even in the late stage, it is possible to share the journey together and make it meaningful right to the very end.

Again, I want to emphasize that Mike and I had nine-and-a-half years together after diagnosis. The first seven years were easier than the last two. But I want you to know that we created many wonderful memories during each and every one of those nine-and-a-half years—memories that our children, grandchildren and I continue to treasure.

Looking back, I now know that the pact we made to stay together as long as possible in our own home was the critical element in determining the quality of our Alzheimer's journey. The details of that pact are described for you in the next chapter.

—————————————— INSIGHTS ——————————————

- Being diagnosed with Alzheimer's is not an imminent death sentence. Statistically speaking, much life lies ahead for you and your loved one after diagnosis.

- I like the saying, "We are living with—not dying from—Alzheimer's."

- Beware of time limits. No one, not even your doctor, can know with certainty how much time you have. As of this writing, there is still no cure for Alzheimer's, but times and treatments are changing and improving even as I write this.

- Have faith, and move forward with your life, knowing that every remaining year can be very meaningful and worthwhile. And remain hopeful that even if a near-term cure is not probable, it is possible.

PART II

~

Preparing Together
for the Road Ahead

CHAPTER 4

MIKE AND I MAKE A DEAL

Not long after the diagnosis,
Mike shared his deepest concern
and greatest fear with me.

AFTER WE RECEIVED THE OFFICIAL DIAGNOSIS and had our immediate questions answered, Mike and I both retreated for a while into a kind of stunned silence.

With the diagnosis, your life has been turned upside down. All your hopes and dreams have been altered, for now you know there is no easy solution to this "little problem" that you had hoped would just go away with the right diet, more exercise, a few crossword puzzles, or a pill.

As time progressed, the diagnosis brought with it a lot of new emotions. We were both doing our best to process this new reality. Down deep, we each had our own separate fears which we were mulling over but not yet ready to verbalize to each other.

Instead of confronting or discussing our biggest fears, we busied ourselves with the obvious practical concerns: reviewing our finances, evaluating our insurance, seeing an attorney, and arranging for Mike to give me Power of Attorney (more on that later). None of these were pleasant tasks. Understandably, Mike resisted addressing them at first, but we eventually agreed to meet them head-on—sooner rather than later—so he could share in the decision-making.

At first, I thought things were going as well as possible under the circumstances. But Mike was obviously angry over the diagnosis and began to be uncharacteristically short with me and grouchy over even the smallest things. I have been told that anger is actually a symptom or expression of other underlying emotions, such as sadness, grief, and disappointment. I think all were present for Mike, but the one I saw most at this point was anger. Yes, I understood why his usual pleasant personality had now become so difficult, but it wasn't easy being at the other end of his frustration. I wondered, was this how it would be throughout the course of his illness? I hoped not.

I THINK WE CAN DO THIS AT HOME

One day while we were working in the yard, Mike was grouchy once again. I wondered what was on his mind. I walked closer to him and he said, quietly but clearly, "I don't want to leave you and our home."

I don't want to leave you and our home! There it was, a simple statement of his greatest fear. It wasn't death or the loss of his physical abilities. Mike's deepest fear and greatest concern was the prospect of eventually having to leave our home and me—to go live in a care facility.

I understood immediately and moved closer. Without much hesitation I said, "I think we can do this at home."

We talked a little more, it was emotional; I don't know exactly what was said in the yard that day. I do know that, by the end of the conversation, Mike's tone of voice and attitude had changed. We had made a deal with each other—a mutual commitment: As long as it was safe for him and for me, Mike and I would live together in our home and make the Alzheimer's journey together. If, for some reason, our stay-at-home plan didn't work, we could always turn to an excellent care facility as our plan B. But for now, we had made a pact to stay together in our home.

"Let's get on with it," he said finally. I wasn't quite certain what that meant to Mike, but I was pretty sure it meant, "Let's not waste any more time on being sad or grumpy; let's get on with enjoying life to the fullest as long as possible."

That was my desire, too. We had made a deal, and I was determined to do my part and more. But somewhere in the back of my mind I heard that persistent voice, asking, "Did I just make a deal that I cannot keep?"

─────────────── **INSIGHTS** ───────────────

- After months of brooding and sadness after the diagnosis, Mike finally got to, "Let's get on with it." That new attitude was so important.

- Moving forward, Mike often said, "There isn't any point in being upset or angry, there isn't anything I can do about it."

- Mike's change in attitude was huge in how we prepared for the Alzheimer's journey ahead and made all the difference in how we continued our next years together. We had both concluded that time had not run out on our dreams and aspirations yet. Instead, our mantra became, "Let's savor every moment."

- In my "couples' relationship" classes I teach parents the importance of being a team and working together to solve problems. Mike and I had done a pretty good job with that over our 35 years together. The question now was, could we continue to do it with a disease like Alzheimer's?

- My greatest fear in this early stage was that we would no longer be a couple at the end of our time together. I now know that, despite Alzheimer's, it is possible to keep your love, friendship and relationship intact right up to the very last day.

CHAPTER 5

DESIGNATING MIKE'S POWER OF ATTORNEY

After hearing Mike's diagnosis,
getting our affairs in order was soon
on my radar, even though it was
not at first on Mike's.

ALL OF US ARE GOING TO DIE SOME DAY, it's a normal part of our shared humanity. Making peace with the knowledge that death is certain can actually make life sweeter by helping us treasure and use the days we still hold in our hands.

Still, most of us would rather not think about death or talk about it—at least not right now. I guess that's just human nature. In fact, many people in western society avoid doing common-sense things such as preparing a living will, or reviewing their life insurance, or even discussing their preference for a memorial service, simply because it's easier to put off the thought of dying.

As we get older, we are reminded more frequently that "now is the time to get your affairs in order." But when something like Alzheimer's comes along, you hear those words with a new urgency. After hearing Mike's diagnosis, getting our affairs in order was soon on my radar, even though it was not at first on Mike's.

In the early stages of Mike's Alzheimer's, I didn't yet know all the things that Mike and I should be thinking about, but I did know that the basics included a Power of Attorney, an updated will, and a Living Will.

You already know what a will is, but you may not be certain about what a Power of Attorney or a Living Will are about, so here's a primer:

A *Durable Power of Attorney* is simply a legal authorization to act on someone else's behalf if that person is ever unable to speak or act for themselves. For example, if Mike assigned me his Power of Attorney, I could then act on his behalf if he could no longer make difficult decisions, or approve legal papers, or competently sign a check on his own.

A *Living Will* is important, too, because it lays out in writing what you wish to happen in the event that you become seriously ill or comatose. If there seems to be no chance of recovery, for example, do you still want the doctors to keep you on life support as long as possible, or would you rather they discontinue all outside help and just let nature take its course?

Obviously, the best time to make those decisions is when you are still clear, healthy and, in legal terms, "of sound mind."

SOONER RATHER THAN LATER

While it's just good common sense to get your affairs in order as soon as possible, that doesn't make it easier for couples to contemplate. I quickly learned that it was not easy for Mike to move forward giving me his Power of Attorney. We came to a stalemate for months. He reasoned that if I had his Power of Attorney, then he should have mine. Hmm, what's wrong with that idea?

A word of caution: By the time Mike finally decided to give me his Power of Attorney, it was almost too late. You see, we needed to have a witness agree that Mike was of "sound mind." Because we waited so long, our attorney told us we were right on the border of when a witness would not be able to confidently agree to that.

What I learned is that it's not necessarily easy giving up your "power" or trusting someone else with your life choices, even if that someone is the one you love most. So I understood what Mike was feeling, and yet I knew this was important to our home-care plan and our future together. Mike also knew, on some level, that this was important and that ultimately he could trust me with this new power.

After months of patient conversations, we were at last at the attorney's office and Mike was ready to sign. Only then did we discover that there are multiple choices when it comes to power of attorney, including medical power, legal power, revocable or irrevocable, and the discussion of advance directive.

Phew! Initially we were thoroughly confused and went away with unsigned papers in hand wondering, what were the right choices for Mike? More time went by, but in the end, he/we decided on a medical and general power of attorney.

FREE TO MOVE ON WITH LIFE

Because Mike made decisions in advance regarding tube feeding, intravenous therapy, and life support equipment, it was easier for me to support his wishes years later at the end of life. I did not have to decide what Mike would want at that time because he had already decided.

Fortunately for me, Mike never discussed the option of ending his own life prematurely. We did not discuss it and, in the end, I did not feel this was something he would want. However, it is interesting to note that Washington State was the second state to pass a Death with Dignity Act, which went into effect in March of 2009.

Working with an attorney to make these cognitive choices together was not the hard part for me. The hard part was thinking of Mike lying in bed some day, nearing the end of his life, and not being able to give him IVs when he could no longer drink.

Truthfully, neither of us wanted to think about what the end of his life would be like. We just knew that once we got our affairs in order, we could go back to focusing on life, love and the future.

────────────── INSIGHTS ──────────────

- With Alzheimer's, judgment and cognitive abilities will be gradually diminishing, so it's important to get your affairs in order sooner rather than later. Mike didn't sign the papers until three years after his diagnosis. Looking back, I now know we were pushing the boundaries and should have done it sooner while Mike was at his clearest.

- If you have Alzheimer's, be sure to give your Power of Attorney to your wife, husband, friend, or family member who you trust to help ensure you have the end of life you choose.

- If you are the partner or caregiver of the person with Alzheimer's, be gentle, patient and clear when discussing these legal issues. Help your loved one understand the wisdom of signing these papers as soon as possible.

- Don't be surprised if signing papers requires you to confront the distress and sadness that Alzheimer's inflicts. However, over time you will discover that having the paperwork in order gives you a certain comfort and freedom from worry.

CHAPTER 6

CALCULATING THE COST OF OUR HOME-CARE PLAN

Our decision to care for Mike at home ultimately saved us countless thousands of dollars.

WHEN SOMEONE YOU LOVE IS DIAGNOSED with a serious illness, you want to do everything in your power to make their life as comfortable and joyful as possible. You'll give them your love, your time, your care and, if necessary, all your earthly possessions. That's exactly how I felt when we learned that Mike had Alzheimer's.

There's an old saying: "If you throw enough money at something, it will eventually go away." But with Alzheimer's that's not true. Mike and I quickly realized that even if we were willing to spend everything we had, this was one thing that was not going to go away. Without careful planning, this disease has the potential of draining virtually anyone's savings or resources.

When Alzheimer's struck, Mike and I had set aside a small nest egg and were living on a modest budget. We had good health insurance along with Mike's Medicare, but we did not have long-term health care insurance. Aside from the equity in our home, we would have no obvious way of paying for Mike to spend years in an Alzheimer's care facility, should that be necessary.

With this in mind, I want to share with you here our thought processes as we made a plan to manage Alzheimer's on our own terms and how we were able to pay for it as we went along.

A DREAM AND A PLAN

When Mike and I made the commitment to care for him at home rather than in a care facility, we had no idea what the outcome would be. All we knew was that we still had a lot of life to live and, despite Alzheimer's, we were determined to stay together forever if possible.

If our commitment to home care didn't work out at some future point, we knew we could always turn to one of several highly regarded Alzheimer's care facilities for help. In a best-case situation, however, our dream was that Mike would be able to live out the rest of his life at our home on Bainbridge Island, with me at his side.

Throughout these pages I will point out some of the many unforeseen blessings that resulted from Mike staying in his own home all those years. It's my belief that living in his own home gave him the kind of purpose, meaning, hope and self-esteem that is difficult to replicate even in a top care facility. Being at home also allowed him to continue relatively seamless relationships with his wife, friends, children and grandchild. And, while I can't prove it scientifically, I'm confident that it ultimately contributed to extending his life, his mobility and even his mental acuity.

As you will see in this chapter, our decision to care for Mike at home also saved us countless thousands of dollars over the course of his nine-and-a-half-year illness.

A LEAP OF FAITH

Right after Mike was diagnosed, we began gathering information about the cost of Alzheimer's. We used the Internet mostly, but also talked with friends, family and other Alzheimer's couples.

Mike and I both wanted him to stay at home if possible, but the responsible thing was to calculate the cost of a good care facility "just in case." So we both agreed that we needed to explore what it would cost to live in a well-regarded care facility.

As you might imagine, Mike was concerned that we would end

up depleting our savings on his Alzheimer's care, and he worried where that would leave me in years to come. I loved him for that. I, on the other hand, was more concerned with how the two of us could afford to continue to live our lives together now, rather than worrying about the distant future.

There were a lot of ifs and unknowns, but we did our homework, estimated the various costs of managing Alzheimer's, and here's what we decided:

Sometimes you have to take a leap of faith and that is what we did. We decided to continue enjoying life, and to make our dreams come true by taking the trips we had planned, and by spending as much quality time as possible with our family and friends.

Instead of living in fear of Alzheimer's, we decided instead to focus on our marriage, to savor each day, and to keep looking forward to every tomorrow. We lived conservatively and responsibly, of course, watching our dollars, using frequent-flyer miles, traveling with family, and staying in inexpensive cottages or campgrounds where we could cook for ourselves.

We also had a backup plan. If it ever turned out that Mike had to be in a care facility and we needed extra dollars, then we would sell our home and give up our other resources too. And I was okay with that, because things are just things.

So we set out to make our dreams come true but continued to keep a wary eye on future costs, knowing always that this disease had the potential to make demands on Mike and me that could possibly bankrupt us, if we weren't vigilant.

HOW WE AFFORDED THE FINAL YEARS

In the "Circle of Friends and Family" chapter ahead I will describe how your circle can hopefully step forward and give you the gift of a few hours of help or care here and there along the way. A morning, a day, or even a weekend—it all adds up through the years to save you and your loved one tens of thousands of dollars.

Because we were managing okay in the early years of Mike's illness (thanks to the help of friends and family) and because Mike did not want someone he did not know providing care for him, I put off hiring a professional caregiver as long as possible. Not paying a caregiver for years was a tremendous help financially. As long as we didn't have the added expense of caregivers, the income from my part-time job paid for our vacations and travel. Once we had to add caregivers, then my income would be used to pay them.

Eventually we did hire two wonderful women to help us in our home. One was a family friend, and the other was a professional caregiver. They made life much easier for Mike and me and, in the end, saved us many thousands of dollars compared to a care facility. (I once calculated that, even after we paid Mike's caregivers, we saved between $4,000 and $6,000 for every month we managed to stay in our home. I'm sure those numbers would be even higher in today's dollars.)

In the last year of Mike's illness our monthly cost for his in-home care rose to $2,000 a month, but this was still a fraction of what a good formal care facility would have cost. Best of all, Mike was still at home surrounded by his loved ones and I was still working a day each week in Seattle and was even able to have a work weekend away from home every six weeks.

While I can't estimate what Alzheimer's will cost you today (it all depends on your individual circumstances), I do know that, if you are wise along the way, there are ways for you to make a huge difference in the ultimate cost. One of those ways, of course, is to care for your loved one in your own home for as long as possible. So make your plan, knowing that you really can manage this disease instead of letting it manage you.

INSIGHTS

- If possible, get a trusted family member or friend to help you make your financial plan. Making financial decisions on your own when you are stressed is no easy matter.

- When Mike was diagnosed, his physician told us that people with Alzheimer's usually live nine years from diagnosis and require two or more years of care in a facility. Benchmarks like these are useful in helping you plan, but don't follow the benchmarks blindly. Mike and I were able to exceed many, if not most, of the typical predictions and expectations for Alzheimer's.

- We did not hire an agency to arrange for Mike's in-home care. If we had, the cost per hour for care would have been more expensive. On the other hand, an agency would have relieved me of doing an individual search for a professional caregiver.

- Some care facilities offer reasonably priced daycare for those with Alzheimer's. This can be a good way to give the primary caregiver an occasional break and is worth looking into.

- Today there is financial aid available for family members who care for loved ones with Alzheimer's at home. Check with your county or state to see if you qualify and refer to the Alzheimer's Association's "MONEY-MATTERS GUIDE" available at ALZ.ORG.

- A reminder to Veterans: Be sure to check on benefits that are available to you including financial assistance for long-term care facilities.

- Hospice paid for Mike's medication, the hospital bed, a Sit-to-Stand lift, a nurse's aid one day a week, and provided immediate care when we needed it. They were just a call away with no cost to us—incredible.

- My top insight, by far, is to go to the Caregiver Center page on the Alzheimer's Association website at www.alz.org and check out the many excellent resources they have to help address the financial and other challenges related to Alzheimer's, including:

- The MONEYMATTERS GUIDE is a detailed booklet outlining financial considerations, from managing and handling bills to health insurance, government benefits and care coverage, and how to get them in order.

- The COMMUNITY RESOURCE FINDER is a comprehensive listing of Alzheimer's and dementia resources, community programs and services that can be filtered to provide access to the most relevant resources.

- The CAREFINDER GUIDE provides information about different care options in the U.S., including tips on communicating with providers.

- The CARE OPTIONS PAGE shows why there is no one-size-fits-all formula when it comes to choosing Alzheimer's care for your loved one. It includes valuable guidance on selecting the most appropriate care setting along with questions to ask when making your decisions.

- The 24/7 HELPLINE is available for those who prefer to discuss these issues with an Alzheimer's Association care expert: 1-800-272-3900.

CHAPTER 7

TO WORK OR NOT TO WORK

*Should you quit your job to be
with your loved one?*

AFTER MIKE AND I AGREED THAT we would tackle Alzheimer's
together at home, I began to wonder if it would be possible to continue working while also providing the kind of care Mike might
need.

I loved my work! It was not just a job to me, it was a calling. For
over 30 years I worked as a self-employed Lamaze childbirth educator which, at the time of Mike's diagnosis, included teaching a weekend retreat in a nearby community once a month. I also worked in
Seattle at Swedish Medical Center, teaching classes for expectant and
new parents. It felt good to make a difference in young couples' lives
and to share in the joy of their children's birth.

At least for now I knew I could continue to work because Mike
could still manage to stay safely at home by himself— but I began to
consider when and how I should prepare for later.

If you are the one providing care for your loved one and you
work outside your home, then you, too, will question if or when
you should quit your job. To help with your decision, here are some
basic questions to consider:

- Is my income essential to our household?
- Can we afford to pay a caregiver when I am away at work?
- How does my current age influence my long-term work plans?
- Would quitting jeopardize my retirement or health insurance?
- Do I have the option of working part time?

- Can I adjust my work hours to accommodate my commitment to my loved one?
- Do I love my work and wish to continue if possible?

And the most important question of all: If I do continue to work, how will it affect quality of life for my loved one with Alzheimer's?

HOW MIKE & I MADE THE DECISION

The first questions were fairly easy for us to answer: I worked part time, my income was helpful rather than required, and our health insurance was not dependent on my work. It was the last question—how would my outside job impact Mike—that was the tough one.

Over time, I concluded that I could continue to work as long as I had three components:

- First, I needed to have the support of Mike and our friends and family.
- Second, I needed to enjoy my work—and I did.
- Third, as Alzheimer's progressed, I would eventually need to find trustworthy professional care for Mike whenever I was away at work.

As it turned out, Mike assured me in multiple conversations that he wanted me to be able to continue to work. He knew I loved my job. He even said at one point that he did not want to be a burden on me and knew I would need my time away. What a lovely gift!

I received the same encouragement from close friends and family. In the early stages of the disease, I would often leave Mike with his good friend Stan when I went to work. It was easy to leave Mike with Stan because they had such a good time together. It was the same with our children. Leaving Mike with them was always easy, for he was their dad and they loved him.

As time went on, and Mike needed continual care, I had to talk to him about bringing professional caregivers into our home. That took some convincing. It was one thing to have Stan, our children, or my sister Patty caring for Mike, but he was not nearly as happy about having a stranger in our home. Patiently, I explained to him, "Mike, this is something you can do for me. If I'm going to continue working, you can help me by allowing someone to care for you while I'm gone." He got it, and did not make a fuss when I went to work. Another Michael gift.

DEALING WITH SEPARATION ANXIETY

Ironically, I was the one who had the most difficulty accepting the idea of leaving Mike at home so I could continue to work. He was my husband, I loved him and now felt very protective of him. More and more, he was vulnerable and I didn't want anything or anyone to harm him. It was such a strange feeling and one that is still hard to explain. Perhaps the closest I can get is to compare it to being protective like a mother is of her child.

I not only had to learn how to leave Mike, but I had to stop thinking about him constantly while at work. I would depart home thinking about Mike, and would have to make a conscious change to focus on work. If I started to forget and wander back to thinking about Mike, then I would remind myself that this was my break, Mike is fine, and I just needed to focus on my work.

It took some time, but I learned to let go whenever Mike was cared for by someone else because I began to see that he was content and happy in their care. When I returned from work, Mike was always happy to see me. With the caregiver's help he would usually tell me about a special place he had been or an experience he had with his caregiver that day. That was reassuring to me.

Working was the right choice for me too. As the disease progressed in future years, Mike's caregivers would encourage me to continue working, knowing that stepping away from Mike's physical care for awhile would surely make a huge difference for me. They were right, of course. When I returned from work, I was glad to be home with Mike not only because I loved him, but because I felt more rested, energized and fulfilled.

Throughout the entire decade of Mike's illness, I continued to assess the feasibility of working and made some adjustments such as changing my hours at the hospital, eliminating a few classes, and decreasing my weekend retreats for parents. Amazingly, I was able to continue to work even in Mike's last year. For this, I remain forever grateful to all of Mike's caregivers. Thank you one and all.

⟿ FROM MY JOURNAL ⟽
JANUARY 2 (YEAR 5)

I just spoke with Patrick and he and Kathleen are gearing up to cover the weekend for me. How lucky I am. I'll look forward to teaching my Getaway class and enjoy some time for me. It is good to know Mike is okay without me and that I am okay without him.

~

The first time I left Mike with others overnight, I wanted to micromanage. Now Pat and Mike buy their groceries and Pat figures it out, so nice for me.

JANUARY 10 (A WEEK LATER)

Patrick and Kathleen are absolutely wonderful with Mike. They enjoy his company and he enjoys them. My two nights away were just right for me. Both Pat and Kathleen have fun with their dad when I am gone. Seems there is lots of laughter for all.

~

These are the good times! I find I don't want to focus too much on where we are heading. We will solve the problems when we get there. For now we need to enjoy each and every day! Time to go back to bed and snuggle with Mike.

- Try to talk together about work as soon as possible—before the disease progresses. Your early conversations will be valuable later.

- Many of my early fears about work turned out to be unfounded, so I gave up worrying. Instead, I simply figured it out from year to year.

- Regardless of what stage he was at in the disease, as long as Mike had good, safe care, everything worked out fine on the work front.

- Remember that the person you love wants to help you. As time goes on, they may not remember or be sure how to help, so it's up to you to inform them clearly: "You can help me and us by doing this . . ."

- Regarding departures and reunions: Research tells us that saying goodbye and greeting your partner is important. So, I always gave Mike a kiss goodbye in the morning when I left for work and then greeted him warmly when I returned. We also had a little chat each night about where I had been and what I had done while I was away that day. When Mike still could, he, too, told me about his day; and when he no longer could, then his caregiver helped him with that.

- Today, I continue to take pleasure in working at Swedish Medical Center, as well as helping and guiding other Alzheimer's couples.

PART III

~

Holding on to
Our Love Story
and Our Dreams

CHAPTER 8

OUR LIFE AND LOVE
BEFORE ALZHEIMER'S

*In every Alzheimer's story there is
also a love story. Hold onto yours,
for it can carry you through the longest days and darkest nights
of your journey.*

WHEN YOU ARE YOUNG AND FALLING IN LOVE, all good things lie ahead, and the last thing on your mind is Alzheimer's. That's the way it once was for Mike and me, many years ago—and here is how we met.

I was nineteen and in the wonder of my years, new at Community College, new at learning about the opposite sex, and in love with the idea of becoming a nurse. My hope was to qualify for the nursing program at Sacramento City College. My plan was to finish the electives first and then see if they might consider this young woman who so wanted to help the world.

While I had seen Mike a few times around campus, my first real memory of him was the day I was struggling to park my stepmother's 1952 Pontiac. Mike waited patiently in his little car while I attempted to shoehorn my big car into a small space. When I gave up, he took the place for his much smaller English Ford. I wondered if he might wait while I parked and walk me to class—and he did. His opening line was, "Do you date short guys?" "Yes," I smiled, and our story began.

Prior to our first date, my dad wanted some information about this young guy. I knew little, except that he was from Montana and had taken a law enforcement class with one of my friends. So my father issued two rules for that first date: do not go out of town, and return early.

We had a noon date, which turned into an all-day date, followed by a movie. First we went to a rodeo in Auburn (out of town, of course) and then a good movie, *Tom Jones*.

We had a wonderful day together. Along the way I learned that Mike was eight-and-a-half years my senior. Unlike me, he had already tasted life, a boy from rural Montana who had dropped out of community college and joined the Army in 1957, the end of the Korean War. After boot camp at Fort Ord in California, he was sent to Seoul, Korea. The years in a foreign country had provided new experiences and maturity.

Mike's father Emil, a miner, and his mother, Micky, divorced when Mike was nine. Mike stayed with his mother who went to work for the military in Oakland, California. Because Mike had too much freedom while his mother was at work, she decided to get him off the streets of Oakland by enrolling him in St. Vincent's School for Boys in San Rafael.

Mike entered my life as an unusual mix. He was street smart and worldly, but also tender and caring. He had the ability to listen and understand, but his colorful vocabulary could be shocking to me. He liked to tell the story that at a young age, the lumberjacks enjoyed teaching him to swear while he sat on the bar top at Del's Bar in Sommers, Montana. Mike was a little rough around the edges, but such a good man inside, and I soon fell in love.

A LITTLE ABOUT ME

My life prior to meeting Mike was checkered with loss. I was born November 30, 1943 in Ely, Nevada. My father, William Martinez, was a good-hearted man. He was devoted to his wife and three daughters, and served for a time in the Nevada State House of Representatives. When I was nine or ten he moved the family to

St. George, Utah, so he could take a job managing a Sprouse-Reitz mercantile store. Little did we know how that move would devastate our family.

In 1952, there were atomic bomb tests done on the Nevada desert, sending toxic clouds over St. George. The long-term health effects are now well-documented. Sadly, my mother was one of many who fell ill. She died of cancer on December 19, 1956 at age 35, leaving behind a husband with three young daughters: Geraldine 15, myself 13, and little sister, Patty, age 4.

I know that losing my mother at a young age played a big role in my desire to become a nurse, and later gave me the ability to stand by Mike in his fight with Alzheimer's. Throughout my mother's illness, I watched as my grandmother, Geraldine, and my father stayed by my mother's side and provided loving care. When we lost our mother, my grandmother and father fought through their own grief to continue caring for my sisters and me. This loving example of "family caring for family" at the end of life would become important when Mike and I lived through his last chapters.

WHEN MIKE AND I BECAME HUSBAND AND WIFE

After graduating from nursing school in 1965, I went to Washington, D.C. to attend a post-graduate program in pediatrics. It was the first time I had lived away from home. Mike's faithful Sunday night phone calls, which I took at the pay phone down the hall, only confirmed that I wanted to spend the rest of my life with him.

I returned to Sacramento and we were married at All Saints Episcopal Church, May 21, 1966. Ours was a typical wedding for the time, about 80 people with cake and coffee in the parish hall. Mike and I honeymooned on the California coast for a week and then started our life together at 9800 Peacock Court in Mountain View, California.

Everything started out great for us. I was a nurse at Stanford Medical Center. Mike went to work for U.S. Customs, first on the waterfront in San Francisco and then as a Special Agent in Los Angeles. Our first child, Patrick Michael, was born a month before we made the move to L.A. Mike and I were in love and completely captivated with our little fellow who arrived with bright red hair.

It was a good time in our lives. Mike was thoroughly involved in his new job, and I was a contented mom. To keep my hand in nursing, I decided to become a certified Lamaze instructor, which eventually became a lifelong love and career for me. Having dinners with friends, play groups, a move to a bigger home, and vacations to Montana filled our life. I look back on those early years of our marriage with such fond memories.

Our second child, Kathleen Marie, was born in the spring of 1974. She arrived with beautiful strawberry blond hair and was pure delight. I was so happy with Kathleen and Patrick that I couldn't see what was waiting for Mike and me right around the corner.

FOR BETTER OR WORSE

Somewhere in the middle of a new home, a new baby, and two demanding careers, Mike and I lost our way. Mike was growing unhappy at work and felt unloved at home. I began to feel under-appreciated and resentful. By the time Kathleen was two, Mike was not only unhappy with work but with our marriage.

Sometimes, by chance or by luck, the right choice is made at the right time. In this case, Mike chose to go to counseling and to stick with our marriage. Two years later we came out the other side in a much better place than we had ever been. I look back now and know that the hard work we did then to save our relationship carried forward and strengthened us for our eventual fight with Alzheimer's.

One other crisis brought us strength: In 1986 Mike accepted a promotion with Customs to be Special Agent in Charge of Internal Affairs for The Northwest Region. We had enjoyed 18 good years in San Pedro, but this new job was in Seattle. While on temporary assignment, Mike discovered beautiful Bainbridge Island, a pleasant thirty-five-minute ferry commute from downtown Seattle, and then a short walk to the Federal building. That's where we decided to make our new home.

Life on Bainbridge Island brought the normal ups and downs, with our children adjusting and me rebuilding my childbirth practice. The crisis came in 1992—out of the blue—when I was diagnosed with breast cancer. The mastectomy and chemotherapy were frightening, to say the least, but ultimately successful. Through it all, Mike remained rock solid, endearing himself to me on a whole new level. I will never forget the day I stood in the bathroom, looking in the mirror, tears welling up in my eyes. As I took off the dressing to look at the incision where my breast had been, Mike gently put his arms around me and said, "You are not your breast."

The office of Internal Affairs was closed in 1988, so Mike ended his career in Washington, D.C., biding his time until he could take early retirement and rejoin his family on Bainbridge Island. The exact date of his retirement was still an unknown. When I flew in to Seattle from a conference in California one day, Mike surprised me at the airport gate.

"I am retired!" he announced with a big grin. Life had never looked better or more promising for Mike and me at that moment. Our encounter with Alzheimer's was still 10 years away.

HOLD FAST TO YOUR LOVE STORIES

"We are the heroes of our own story," wrote author Mary McCarthy. That sentiment takes on special meaning for every couple who braves Alzheimer's together.

Little did we know during the early years of dating and then marriage that Mike and I were creating the chapters of our own ongoing Love Story. Later on, those unique experiences we shared— through good times and bad—would help carry us through the final chapters of our life together with grace and courage. Here's how it worked:

Perhaps like you, over our 40-plus years of marriage, Mike and I lived through many memorable moments and experiences, some romantic, some hilarious, some beautiful, some tragic, and some filled with adventure. When Alzheimer's shadow touched our lives, we could look back on those memories and savor every little chapter of our Love Story. No discussion was necessary. In certain situations, we would simply glance at each other, or raise an eyebrow, or say a word, and instantly we found ourselves reliving an earlier and more pleasant part of our life together.

Later, as Mike's memory began to diminish, our Love Story was in jeopardy, but we did not just let it slip away. We kept our Love Story alive by telling it to each other as long as possible, and by sharing our story often and in detail with others, especially those who had lived through our story with us. When Mike could no longer tell our stories himself, I became the storyteller. And oh, yes, it was time to bring out the photos!

During the later stages of Alzheimer's, our Love Story would become especially important, for it grounded us and allowed us to remember and revisit the good times we had together as we continued our marriage, friendship and love through the last chapters of the disease.

So, whether you are in the early stage, the mid stage, or the later stage of Alzheimer's I encourage you and your partner to cling to your Love Story too. Remember to share it again and again as you continue your journey, for it can carry you through the longest days and darkest nights. Your Love Story will make you laugh, and sometimes make you cry, and both are okay—especially while living with Alzheimer's.

I have enjoyed sharing some of Mike's and my Love Story with you, and I will share more in the pages ahead. Not all, of course, for some stories are just for Mike and me.

CHAPTER 9

KEEPING THE SPARK ALIVE

*After the diagnosis, Mike and I both
had fears about where our marital
relations might be heading.*

A FEW MONTHS AFTER MIKE WAS DIAGNOSED he came to me
with concern in his eyes. He had heard on the radio that people
with Alzheimer's may enjoy sex at first, but then eventually lose
interest. He was concerned that this might happen to him and wanted
to talk with me about this new fear.

I listened to Mike's worry and told him that I hoped that would
not be the case and assured him that he had always been a good
lover and that I was optimistic that would continue. Then we agreed
that we were both currently enjoying our love life and that there
was no point in worrying about something that was not yet a problem. If it ever became a problem, then we would figure it out.

Still, I had my own fears about where our marital relations might
be headed with Alzheimer's. I had seen reports of a married Alzheimer's patient falling in love with another patient at their care facility.
And, in other cases, people acting out sexually or saying inappropriate things in public.

Mike and I typically talked about our fears, but on this fall morning it did not seem right to give him one more worry. So I kept my
fears to myself and put them in the category of "we will wait and see."

SEX AND INTIMACY WITH ALZHEIMER'S

Much has been written about the all too common marital problems or sexual issues associated with Alzheimer's. But very little

has been written about couples like Mike and me who remained deeply in love and were able to enjoy intimacy right to the end. That is what I would like to tell you about here.

According to the Alzheimer's Association, the most commonly encountered problems in intimacy and sexuality are:

- misidentification of intimate partners
- fear/paranoia around intimacy
- accusations of infidelity
- caregiver loneliness
- excessive demand for sex

With Mike and me none of these issues came to pass. Throughout the entire nine-and-a-half years of his illness, Mike did not lose his desire for me, or fall in love with someone new, or make demands for affection, or say things that were inappropriate.

To the contrary: Mike's concern for me, his frequent gestures of appreciation, his tender eye contact, and his ability to remember our love story when I reminded him continued year after year. And my feelings for him followed the same path, defying the daily frustrations of Alzheimer's and bringing us even closer together in love and affection as time went on.

Research tells us that a good relationship is the key to a good love life, not vice versa. I believe that is true for Alzheimer's couples too. Mike and I both nurtured our relationship even when Alzheimer's sorely tested our patience with each other. We were not overly surprised, then, when our intimacy continued long beyond the usual expectations for Alzheimer's couples.

As unlikely as it may seem, Mike was sexually active until age 75, and we even made love just months before he started hospice care. I tell you this to assure you that love, yearning and beauty can continue to grow and survive even in the shadow of Alzheimer's. I hope this is hopeful and encouraging for you and your loved one, and for Alzheimer's couples everywhere.

As you will see in my journal notes below, it's not the big romantic dinners or expensive cruises that kept the spark of love alive for Mike and me. For us, as for all couples, it really was the little daily things: A tender touch, a thoughtful smile, a sincere thank you or I love you. These are the things that help chase the Alzheimer's shadow away and keep the lamp of love burning brightly.

⟿ FROM MY JOURNAL ⟽

YEAR ONE

JANUARY

Mike couldn't sleep for a few nights, said he is thinking of a lot of things. Told me he has nightmares about not being able to take care of me. We continue to fall more in love, as we know our time is short. We are both optimistic that we have time.

NOVEMBER

Mike tells me daily, "I love you . . . you feel so soft" . . . and (my favorite) "goodnight sweetheart." Sex is good for us right now. Mike is pleased with how well everything is working. He said, "I don't think we have ever been more tuned into each other." Someplace he read that sex is good for Alzheimer's people and then it goes away. Maybe these are the good times!

YEAR TWO

DECEMBER

My 60th birthday was special—Mike made dinner reservations at Ruby's. "Table with a view at 7 PM." Very special that he planned ahead. Mike took two hours to get ready—he said it felt like a first date to him. He looked cute in plaid pants, green V-neck sweater and dress shoes. Lovely night!

YEAR THREE

AUGUST

*I had a bone scan done. It was scary for me. The tech who gives
radioactive dye began to strap me down and told Mike he couldn't
stay. I said, "No straps and I want my husband back."
Mike touched my arm and talked to me about Mt. Brook. At one
point he growled and showed me he was my protector;
made me laugh. I love him!*

YEAR FOUR

APRIL

*Our 39th Anniversary. We celebrated early in Victoria, Canada.
Things I want to remember:
–A kiss on the ferry as we docked in Victoria.
–Arm around me on top of the double-decker bus.
–Buying "floral" plates for our 39th anniversary. (Mike liked all
different flowers, so that is what we got.)
–A man at the Parliament building telling Mike to remember there
is a dining room in the building. Mike said, "Trust me on this,
I am not the one to remind her." Oh we laughed!
Mike and I had a wonderful time.*

YEAR SIX

JANUARY

*A few days ago Mike looked at my wedding rings and said they
were pretty. He asked, "Where did go get them." I told him and he
looked like it was new information to him.*

Note to reader: When Mike asked about my wedding rings, I told
him that he had given them to me years ago. Then I clicked our
rings together and said, "We are married; these are our wedding
rings—we go together." Mike seemed to understand because his
eyes opened wide and his face brightened.

YEAR SEVEN

MARCH

*We had a lovely little dance in the kitchen to the tune of "Always".
Then, as we got into bed Mike told me we should take dancing
lessons. I told him that would be fun.*

MAY

*Mike gave me a hug and "I love you!" as we stood next to the bed.
He frequently says "Have I given you a kiss?"
I always say no and get a kiss.*

YEAR EIGHT

MAY

*Mike continues to enjoy walking up the driveway to get the
newspaper and mail. This morning he made a second trip up the
driveway to pick a dandelion for me. Sometimes he says "Did I tell
you I love you?" Another favorite is "hey" and then a kiss.*

YEAR NINE

MAY

*Friday was our 44th anniversary. We awoke early, stayed in bed
and talked about when we got married and memories of our hon-
eymoon. Next thing I knew we were making love.*

THE LAST TIME MIKE AND I MADE LOVE

The day of our 44th wedding anniversary was special for Mike and
me, in several ways. Through the years, our anniversary had always
been a pleasant day for us. Usually we went out for a luxurious dinner or took a little trip, but now Mike was in his ninth year of Alzheimer's. What could we do? Well, I could still plan a special meal
at home and get a romantic DVD and I did just that.

Reminiscing about the day we were wed was something I often did with Mike. Whenever he was uncertain about my wedding

rings or of something in the past, I brought out the photo album and brought him back to pleasant old memories of our lifelong love story.

Now, on this particular morning of our 44th anniversary, we sat on our bed, smiling and talking of our wedding day, and our life together, and of the pleasure of being married all these years. The next thing I knew we were making love and enjoying the closeness that only a long relationship can engender.

Mike and I had steadfastly enjoyed our lovemaking throughout the many years of his illness, but it had become less frequent toward the end, and I was pretty sure this would be the last time we shared the intimate moment together. And it was.

But even though sex had come to an end for Mike and me that day, our lovemaking continued in the form of snuggling, holding hands, a shared smile, eyes meeting eyes, or a tender kiss right up until just days before he died.

Some would say that the sweet morning of our 44th anniversary was the last time we made love, but I say we made love right up to the very last day of Mike's life.

INSIGHTS

- Again, Mike and I were committed to managing Alzheimer's together at home instead of a care facility. Living at home as husband and wife made it easier for us to maintain a close, loving, physical relationship to the very end.

- The fact that Mike was able to make love with me so late in the disease is hopeful—but it wasn't the most important thing to Mike and me. Sex or no sex, the important thing for us was to maintain the love that originally brought us together, long before Alzheimer's entered our lives.

- The simple loving things that worked for us will hopefully work for you and your loved one, too, including:

  √ Tell the one you love how special they are.

  √ Tell him or her you are proud of them for managing this difficult disease.

√ Bring out your old photos again and again, and use them to tell your loved one the familiar stories of your romance.

√ Remember to praise and appreciate your partner in your everyday life.

√ Talk openly about your love life and remind your partner what you like.

√ Remind your partner of the good times and romantic memories you share from years past.

√ Despite Alzheimer's, continue to make time for dating and romance, no matter how simple your dates may eventually become.

√ Plan your intimate moments (mornings worked best for us).

√ To learn more about sexuality and Alzheimer's, go to the Alzheimer's Association website: www.alz.org

CHAPTER 10

FULFILLING OUR
TRAVEL DREAMS

*Mike and I still had dreams of trips
to faraway places and knew that, if
we were ever going to realize those
dreams, we better get a move on.*

THIS MIGHT SURPRISE YOU but Mike and I managed to travel just fine for years after Mike's diagnosis, and we had many good times and adventures together.

Needless to say, a lot depends on where you are in the disease process and what your previous view has been on travel. If you never liked to travel before Alzheimer's, you probably won't like it now. But couples who have traveled happily in the past should feel optimistic about more travels to come.

As for Mike and me, we discovered that our decision to keep on traveling came with unexpected benefits. Planning a trip did more than just keep our previous travel dreams alive. It gave us something new and exciting to look forward to. It gave us an opportunity to visit distant friends and family. Best of all, a trip to a new place helped take our focus off Alzheimer's and allowed us to just be us again.

In this chapter I'll recount a few details of what we did and how we did it on each trip because I want you to see how traveling changed for us as Mike's Alzheimer's progressed. My hope is that, if you are in the early or middle stages of Alzheimer's, our travel experiences will give you the confidence to consider making plans for your own adventures.

YOU HAVE TO GO TO KNOW

Early in our marriage, Mike and I were not world travelers by any means. We did manage two memorable trips to Europe when we were young—one to Germany in the 1980s and another to visit my sister and her family in Italy. Those two trips made us want to see and do more. As the old saying goes, "You can't sit home and see the world; you have to go to know."

When our kids were young, our dreams of traveling to other countries were put on hold. Instead, we acquired our beloved VW camper and managed to travel much of the U.S. in it, including annual trips to Montana to see Mike's family.

When Alzheimer's arrived at our door in 2002, we still had dreams of trips to faraway places and knew that, if we were ever going to realize those dreams, we better get a move on—and we did just that. Despite Alzheimer's, we averaged at least one good trip every year or two. Here are some of the places we went and what we learned along the way.

OUR TRIP TO AUSTRALIA AND NEW ZEALAND
(THE SAME YEAR MIKE WAS DIAGNOSED)

Topping our dream list was a trip to Australia to see our niece Trisha in Brisbane. Visiting Australia is an amazing experience for anyone, but with Alzheimer's there might be a few adventures we could do without.

Making a major trip like this right after you've been diagnosed with Alzheimer's may seem like a crazy idea to some, but we had family there, so we felt we could count on help should we need it.

We discovered that Mike could handle the backpack, which carried his CPAP, but he was not good at keeping track of luggage. That left it up to me to manage the two suitcases on wheels, as well as keep track of Mike. At this point in the illness, he could still navigate pretty well on his own, but I always needed to be vigilant that he did not walk off in the wrong direction.

One of my favorite memories of Australia is a young koala bear snuggled on Mike's shoulder. We waited for some time to have our turn with this little fellow. When Mike's turn came, he was so gentle and so proud when the attendant praised him for his tender touch.

We ventured on to Northern New Zealand's outer edge in a small plane with Mike buckled in up front with the pilot. The view was spectacular as we looked down at high snow-covered peaks. It made me so happy to see Mike grinning ear to ear. He loved an adventure, and we were certainly having one. We came down out of the sky to a beautiful bay, where a small boat awaited with a guided tour of the inlet. Incredible!

⟿ FROM MY JOURNAL ⟵

New Zealand and Australia were wonderful for both Mike and me. It slowed life down for us. A few trouble spots: forgot some meds, plug for CPAP incorrect, lost credit card. Could have lost Mike at the airport or in downtown area, too, but we did fine. Trisha was wonderful!

OUR TRIP ACROSS CANADA
(ONE YEAR AFTER MIKE WAS DIAGNOSED)

Our trip across Canada in our trusty VW camper was truly amazing. We had a wonderful time in the Maritime Provinces, New Brunswick, Nova Scotia, and Prince Edward Island. The trip ended with seeing our friends, the Davenports, and meeting our daughter Kathleen and son Patrick in Maine, followed by a six-day drive home to Bainbridge Island. And we did it all, despite Alzheimer's!

⟿ FROM MY JOURNAL ⟵

I now look back and cannot believe we did it. I did all the driving, 13,000 miles. Our routine was pretty easy: Mike pumped gas, washed windows, and set up the camper. I drove and cooked. It was easy because I always knew where he was.

⁓

Mike shopped on his own at an Army Surplus store in Winnipeg and found a port-a-potty for our camper. At Fundy National Park, he got lost. Restrooms were behind us, but we pulled in the campground at night and got turned around. After 30 minutes, I was ready to go looking. But he figured it out himself by going back to the entry of the park and found our campsite!

OUR TRIP TO RENO AND LOS ANGELES (TWO YEARS AFTER MIKE WAS DIAGNOSED)

Going to Reno and Southern California at this stage in Mike's illness was so fun for both of us. This was not a trip to see the sights, it was a journey to visit treasured friends and family, many of whom Mike would probably never see again.

It was good to go back and see our old community that we cherished for 18 years, including the schools, our favorite grocery store, and family home. But most of all it was good to share memories with our old friends, for they had been like family for the first years of our marriage and our children's lives.

We laughed a lot with our friends and shed a few tears, too, knowing we were experiencing some of our last memories with Mike.

⇝ FROM MY JOURNAL ⭒

Smooth flight to Reno, saw family and then drove to Los Angeles and saw the San Pedro gang. Spent a pleasant 5 days then went north to see Bill and Kathy and on to Sue and Ray's.

⁓

Monday we drove over snowy Donner Pass and celebrated my 61st birthday in Reno with the family. We flew home Tuesday on my birthday. Pat cooked spaghetti, and Kathleen brought a carrot cake. Lovely birthday! Mike and I are so lucky to be surrounded by good friends and family.

OUR TRIP TO IRELAND
(THREE YEARS AFTER MIKE WAS DIAGNOSED)

The trip to Ireland was a long-held dream of Mike's, and dreams deserve to come true—especially when you happen to have Alzheimer's. We made the trip this time with our two children and their partners. As always, I wondered in advance, "Can we actually do this?" It turned out that we could and we did—and I continue to treasure those fond Irish memories and still love watching the DVD our son made of the trip.

⤚ FROM MY JOURNAL ⤙

Ireland—what a special time. We were gone an entire month. Patrick, Kathy, Kathleen, and Sam joined us. It made it all perfect. We stayed in only a few different locations: eleven days in an apartment in Dublin; one night in Waterford; a week in a little cottage near the Cliffs of Moher; four nights in Limerick; four nights in Killarney. And one last night back in Dublin. Six different locations in 30 nights was just right for Mike.

⁓

Discovered early meals better than late for Mike. Long stops in bathroom airport made me worry that Mike would not make the flight, but no problem. Mike got off the city bus once without us, but Sam and Kathleen were on it and got him back. Mike was an excellent traveler and made me realize we can still go.

MIKE'S SOLO TRIP TO SACRAMENTO
(FOUR YEARS AFTER HE WAS DIAGNOSED)

Prior to Alzheimer's, Mike enjoyed taking occasional solo trips to Sacramento to visit his good friend Herb and his wife Pat. Now, four years after diagnosis, he decided to make the trip again.

I worried, "Can he do this by himself?" But thanks to the loving care of Herb and Pat, who made sure he had his pills on time, kept good track of him, and filled his visit with laughter, Mike managed just fine, and came home to me safe and happy.

Mike had a most excellent trip to Sacramento. I continue to wonder when it will be the last. I alerted Alaska Airlines that Mike might need help, but it turned out that he actually needed very little.

OUR TRIP TO ALASKA
(FIVE YEARS AFTER MIKE WAS DIAGNOSED)

We had a wonderful trip to Alaska to visit with my sisters Patty and Gerrie, and to attend my nephew Paul's wedding to Jenny.

We built in a few extra vacation days and went to Chena Hot Springs with Patty and Gerrie. We got our own little cabin and I cherish the memory of the night he surprised me with the gift of a delightful dress watch. He had thoughtfully picked the watch out for me with Patty's help. That night he proudly pointed out the hearts and little diamonds on it.

OUR TRIP TO COLORADO SPRINGS
(SIX YEARS AFTER MIKE WAS DIAGNOSED)

Even this far into our Alzheimer's journey, Mike and I managed another very significant (and fun!) road trip. This time it was a long and scenic drive to Colorado Springs for my niece Allison's wedding. All went well again, thanks as always to having family at the end of the road.

Two favorite memories: Mike dancing with Allison and the children at the wedding reception. And then later going on the dramatic cog railway ride up Pike's Peak.

I'm proud to say that Mike and I were able to attend three beautiful weddings in three years: Jenny and Paul in Alaska; Kathleen and Sam in Washington; and Allison and Kyle in Colorado. Despite Alzheimer's, we made them all!

OUR TRIP TO MAUI
(SEVEN YEARS AFTER MIKE WAS DIAGNOSED)

I have very fond memories of our trip to Maui, Hawaii, for it was our last big trip. On this particular adventure, I knew we needed to keep our itinerary as uncomplicated as possible, so I arranged for a condo where we could settle in, cook our own meals, and easily walk places.

It was just two years before Mike would no longer be with us, and yet here we were in Hawaii, still enjoying the palm trees and the beaches and making memories. It was both amazing and heart-warming, for this is not what I had been led to expect.

Like all our previous trips, I was initially worried about how things would unfold on Maui. But it turned out that all I needed was a little faith in Mike and a little courage (and planning) on my part, and it was not only possible, it was priceless.

⇀ FROM MY JOURNAL ↽

We had a wonderful trip to Maui with Kathleen, Sam and baby Riley. Flight went well both coming and going.

Maui memories:

- *Mike smiling at Riley, and Riley smiling back as she played with her mobile.*
- *Beautiful sunsets from our condo*
- *Pineapple tour with Mike*
- *Drink with Mike at the Ritz*
- *Mike in the pool with Kathleen and Sam*
- *Easter Sunday at the "open wall" Episcopal church*
- *Our walk across the golf course and Mike stopping to give me a kiss and saying "I love you."*

~

From my perspective the Maui trip was perfect. I loved the

*beautiful (but expensive) condo and ease of
walking places with Mike or by myself.*

*After we got home, I knelt by the bed and told Mike how great he
did with everything on the trip. I said to him, "Everything was different for you: bathroom, car, stairs, table, and food." Then I said:
"Everything was different but me." At the same time he said "but
my wife." We laughed at our shared thought.*

INSIGHTS

- Soon after Mike was diagnosed, someone advised us to keep things as normal as possible for as long as possible—and travel helped us do that. Travel was something we liked to do together so we kept it as part of our life as long as possible.

- The journal entries for our trips are short and without much detail. When we traveled, I did not think to take a journal with me; I wish I had. But, in reality, I was way too busy to write much.

- The hard part during any trip was that, when we were on our own, I had to be vigilant for Mike 24/7. At home, I could count on help from family and friends, and look forward to quiet times in the afternoon when Mike rested.

- Would I do those trips all over again? Absolutely! However, I could not have made any of these trips without the backup of family and friends.

- Family provided: conversation, another set of hands to help with Mike, eyes to be sure all was safe, and help with unanticipated challenges.

- I am glad Mike and I continued to build memories together after his diagnosis. For today Mike is even more vividly remembered by the stories we created together and with others through our travels.

- While not everyone will be able to travel in the later stages of Alzheimer's as Mike and I did, I expect that many more could if they only believed it was possible and did a little planning.

- Despite Alzheimer's, I encourage you to talk with each other, find out what is important to you, get on with your dreams and have fun building memories. And if your dreams include travel, then you might just be able to do that too.

CHAPTER 11

HOW LOVE CAN TRIUMPH OVER ALZHEIMER'S

*As Mike's illness gradually
progressed, some were surprised by
our ability to continue on as husband
and wife, despite the discouraging
limitations of the disease.*

WHEN I FIRST BEGAN WRITING THIS BOOK, I asked friends
and family to send me their memories of the times they spent with
Mike and me during his illness. Looking back, there are two things
that seem to stand out for most people, and I think both of them are
surprising and hopeful for all Alzheimer's couples.

First, even though Mike's memory and physical abilities grew
more and more impaired as time went on, he never completely lost
the core of who he was. In other words, Mike never stopped being
Mike, and his friends and family never stopped relating to him as
the Mike we all knew and loved.

Second, throughout the entire nine-and-a-half years, right up to
the very last weeks before he died, Mike and I were able to maintain
our close connection as husband and wife. In truth, we were able to
consciously express our love and appreciation for each other, and
continue pursuing life, long after conventional wisdom said our ongoing relationship should have ended. Even later, when the disease
had robbed Mike of his ability to speak or move, I never gave up on
communicating with him, and he never gave up on communicating
with me.

From the day he was first diagnosed, it just seemed natural to continue reaching out to Mike, and I was not surprised when he responded to my words or my touch with loving gestures of his own. Still, our friends and family seemed baffled at times by our ability to carry on as husband and wife, despite all the discouraging limitations of the disease. Here is an example from our dear friend Claudia:

RECALLING HOW ROSALYS
LOVED AND HONORED MIKE

BY CLAUDIA KREIS

"I visited with Rosalys and Mike on several occasions after Mike was diagnosed with Alzheimer's. Each time my heart sang as I observed Rosalys tenderly engaging Mike.

Later, when I went to see Rosalys and Mike during the last months of his life, I discovered something truly unexpected for that late stage. He was still Mike! He could not walk and had lost most of his capacities but he was still Mike. We even danced to music he loved—he in his wheelchair, and Rosalys, Marilyn and me holding his hands and swaying.

It seems to me that what Rosalys did with such systematic devotion was to constantly remind Mike of their special connection. She would show him their wedding rings, or gently remind him of all the good things he had done for his family through the years.

Mike and Rosalys' loving relationship continued to the end. I am convinced it was because of the unceasing communication between them. Even at the very end, here was Rosalys tenderly talking to Mike about their relationship, and here was Mike somewhere in the darkest recesses of his mind, responding to the constant reassurance and friendship from his beloved wife."

Love, Claudia

I am forever thankful to Claudia, Marilyn and other friends and family who witnessed what seemed so natural to me and yet so surprising to them. I fear that many might doubt what happened, and yet I know what Claudia and so many others observed was true. Namely, that despite the severity of his Alzheimer's, Mike was somehow able to stay connected with me and those he loved to the very end, and he surpassed our expectations and preconceived notions in several other ways too.

What does this tell you? It tells you and every other couple who is experiencing this big bully of a disease that we may be giving too much power to Alzheimer's. Perhaps when two people are fiercely bound in love and loyalty as a couple, they are able to deal with this disease together in ways that one person could never do alone. It is not a given, therefore, that your mutual love will be lost, all memories wiped away, feelings for others forgotten, or that the very core of who your loved one is will be swept away by this disease.

I think this is especially true when Alzheimer's couples are living in their own home. Because we lived at home together, things stayed roughly the same for Mike from day to day and from year to year. Old friends stopped by, neighbors came in for a chat, our children visited, and Mike and I even provided care for our granddaughter one day a week.

Staying in our home helped Mike know where he was: his things were always in the same place, the photos of family members stayed on the walls, and our bedroom remained ours for cuddling, laughter and affection. I know this was all comforting and inspiring for Mike and surely contributed to his staying connected to his friends and family and the world.

NEVER GIVE UP ON YOUR LOVED ONE

I learned first-hand that the little things Mike and I did at home as a couple made a huge difference for him and for us. And I'm hopeful and confident that most, if not all, of the things we did you can do too.

First and foremost, make it a rule that you will never give up on your loved one. By this, I mean never let the worsening symptoms of Alzheimer's trick you into thinking that your loved one has drifted into an unconscious or uncaring state and is no longer "there" with you.

Shakespeare wrote, "Love adds a special seeing to the eye," and this beautiful thought has special meaning to Alzheimer's couples. With love you can look beyond your partner's apparent limitations and see the light that still glows inside. Rather than look at all the imperfections or shortcomings brought on by Alzheimer's, love watches for any signs of awareness and affection. Love sees not just what your friend and partner has lost with this disease, but all the qualities and possibilities that are still left.

From the very beginning of the disease, keeping Mike connected to me, our home, and our family was not so difficult after all. I just had to continue treating him like my loving husband, just as I had done for so many years. Alzheimer's did not get to take that away from him or from me. I did it consciously and faithfully. As Claudia wrote above, I did not slip into thinking that Mike was not there. I interacted with him just as I always had, because he was still my husband, my partner, and my dearest friend.

As I've mentioned elsewhere in the book, I frequently used our wedding rings to serve as a favorite reminder that we were connected in a special way. Clicking our rings together, showing him our wedding album and sharing our love story all helped Mike remember who he was and that he and Rosalys went together as a team.

As his ability to engage with others declined in the mid-to-later years, I never talked to others about Mike as if he wasn't present in the room, or as if he wasn't capable of understanding what I was saying. If possible, I moved to his physical level when talking with others, sitting next to him, rather than standing and talking above him. At family gatherings I engaged him with frequent touches, nodding to him, telling his stories to others for him, and drawing him into the conversation at frequent intervals.

None of this was particularly difficult because, after all, this was my husband who I loved. We had walked together in life for 45 years and now it was time to stay by his side and continue to give him the dignity and affection that we all deserve, especially when life plays a dirty trick like Alzheimer's on us.

MIKE DID HIS PART TOO

Some might say that Mike was extraordinary and not the typical person with Alzheimer's, but I disagree. Mike was an everyday, good-hearted guy from Montana who grew up in a less-than-ideal situation and knew how to make the most of the cards that were dealt to him. And while he could not beat the disease in the end, he showed us through the years that love really can triumph over Alzheimer's by dramatically improving the quality of the journey.

In the early years of his illness, Mike showed his appreciation with a sincere thank you, a hand pat, a little smile, or a loving look that could make my eyes water. But even toward the very end there were always little signs that he still loved me and was still with me. A calculated movement of his lips, a lingering look, a little smile we shared of a past memory, a raised brow, a wrinkle between his eyes when concerned for me, a smile of pleasure about something I did, or a little pucker of his lips for a kiss. Yes, love adds a special seeing to the eyes. To stay connected with Mike, all I had to do was watch carefully for these little heartfelt signs, respond to them, and never disregard them.

So, as time goes on, never give up on your loved one, and always treat him or her with dignity. Just because your loved one can no longer communicate as clearly as before, don't assume that they are not right there with you, taking everything in. It is our job to be open to them and love them just as when they could respond more fully and naturally in their pre-Alzheimer's days.

INSIGHTS

- We now know that those who come out of a coma have often been far more aware of what was taking place around them than we realized. I can't help but wonder if something like that is happening with our perceptions of people with severe Alzheimer's. They may be much more aware than we give them credit for.

- Look to your partner's eyes. A newborn child knows the mother by sight, sound, smell, and touch, and yet they cannot express their feelings with words; it is only in their eyes that we see all that's happening in their inner world.

- Mike decided early on that he was not going to be miserable and grumpy about his Alzheimer's diagnosis, and he was true to his word. His positive attitude made a difference in all that we did together for nearly 10 years. So, to those with Alzheimer's: you need to do the best you can to manage this disease so that you, too, can make a difference for the one you love.

- It is fair to say that the disease process is different for everyone, but I now argue that we give Alzheimer's too much credit. I believe the emotional state is a combination of the environment and the disease, and that Alzheimer's couples can have a tremendous effect on the quality of their journey by what they do and how they do it as a couple. This is true in the early going, as well as in the later stages.

- Some believe that, at a certain point in time, a person with Alzheimer's no longer has the ability to know who they are, where they are, or carry the memories of yesterday or today. I never felt that was true for Mike, and I will believe forever that Mike and I were able to diminish the severity of his Alzheimer's by confronting the disease together as a loving couple and team.

CHAPTER 12

WEDDING RINGS HAVE
THEIR STORIES

*Mike's plain white gold band now
resides on a simple chain. I wear
it when I feel weak and want to be
strong, or when I am enjoying a
special celebration or memory.*

As you go through your Alzheimer's journey together, you can expect that your wedding rings will take on new significance. They are, after all, the tangible symbol of a lifelong commitment to each other.

As time goes on, wedding rings hold more and more stories because your rings have been with you through thick and thin, for better or worse, in sickness or in health. That's the way it was for Mike and me.

I love my rings. One is a simple emerald cut diamond, and the other a plain white gold band. I rarely took them off in our 45 years of marriage. Mike, on the other hand, was not a jewelry guy. He chose not to wear his matching band, at least not in the early years of our marriage. But, as you are about to see, that changed as time went on.

I remember the day I got my ring just as clearly as if it was yesterday. Mike and I had talked of marriage and made the final decision while I was at a three-month nursing program in Washington, D.C. We had even discussed the style and color of the ring I would like, and I was confident that when I returned home Mike would give me an engagement ring.

Sure enough, Mike picked me up at the airport, with a little ring box sitting on the dashboard. As he drove he said, "Open it," so I did and there was the simple diamond ring we had talked about. It was a little larger then I expected. Mike explained that his aunt and uncle had helped him order it from a jewelry catalog. Receiving the ring from the dashboard as Mike drove along wasn't very romantic but, well, that is just how it happened.

The ring was lovely, but not yellow gold as we had talked about. I gently mentioned that it was not yellow gold but then said, "White will be fine," and it was.

I grew to love my rings, some days more than others. There was the time our marriage was falling apart, and I was not very happy with either Mike or the rings that were supposed to be the symbol of our love. The rings came off then for a month or so, but Mike and I weathered the storm and they went back on.

A NICE SURPRISE

As I mentioned earlier, wedding rings have stories, and this is one of ours: long before Mike's Alzheimer's diagnosis, my artist friend Amy asked if she could do a painting of me for a portrait exhibit she was creating. I agreed and we soon had a portrait of me hanging above the stairs that led to the family room. A few years later when my birthday rolled around, I asked Mike to have Amy do a portrait of him, too, so we could both hang on the wall together. After a little encouragement, he agreed. It was not really his thing, but he would do it for me as my birthday gift.

When Mike's portrait was finished, Amy brought it to the house for a little unveiling ceremony. She made me wait in the kitchen while she hung his portrait next to mine. When I was finally called in to see the painting, I was so surprised. The first thing I noticed was that Mike had his wedding ring on in the portrait. How thoughtful of him. I had not seen that ring in years; I wasn't even sure that he knew where it was.

"Mike wore his ring!" I said in disbelief. Amy smiled and said, "No he told me about it and asked me to paint it on his finger because he knew you would like that." What a nice birthday surprise that was.

Time rolled by. Although Mike's wedding ring was always there in the portrait for all to see, he still refrained from wearing it in everyday life. He explained that he couldn't really wear a ring while working on cars, or while pursuing certain cases in his job as a federal agent. I accepted his reasons, but it still made me feel a little wistful.

Then one day, after he retired and just a few years before his Alzheimer's diagnosis, Mike did a sudden turnaround. He announced to me that he now wanted his wedding ring on. We went hunting for it together and finally found it—on a bookshelf in a little wooden box that had a secret panel in it. From that day on, Michael wore his wedding ring, even all through the illness, until the day he died. That meant a lot to me.

When Mike was in the last months of his illness, I vowed to remember that I would be the one to take the wedding ring off his finger. I would safely remove Mike's ring when he died, but not before.

Mike's plain white gold band now resides on a simple chain with a heart-shaped charm containing a little photo of him that my daughter so thoughtfully gave to me. I no longer need to always have it by my side, but I do wear it when I feel weak and want to be strong, or when I am enjoying a special celebration or memory.

Yes, wedding rings hold stories and I still hold the stories of Mike and me close to my heart.

PART IV

~

Forming Our Circle
of Support

CHAPTER 13

TELLING OUR FRIENDS THAT MIKE HAS ALZHEIMER'S

*Here's how some of our dearest
friends reacted to the news.*

ALZHEIMER'S HAS A WAY OF deepening some friendships while dampening others—and I've learned that's okay, it's understandable. Some friends simply seem to be better equipped to deal with the intrusion of Alzheimer's than others.

Fortunately for Mike and me, most of our closest friends and family rallied around us from the moment they first heard of the diagnosis. One such couple—Margaret and Mike Gaines—lives in California, but were always willing to jump on a plane to come keep our friendship strong through all the years Mike and I battled this disease.

In Margaret's own words (below) she describes what it was like for her and her husband to hear that Mike had Alzheimer's. I remain forever grateful for her and her husband's steadfast friendship through the years—and for similar support from other dear friends and family.

WHEN I FOUND OUT THAT MIKE HAD ALZHEIMER'S
BY MARGARET GAINES

One day our old friends Mike and Rosalys Peel invited my husband Mike and me to their home. I remember feeling an unusual sense of urgency in this particular invitation.

When we arrived at Mike and Rosalys' home, the four of us gathered around the table out on the deck. It was a beautiful day on Bainbridge Island, but something was obviously about to happen.

Moments later a serious tone came over Mike's voice as he told us there was a reason he had asked us to visit. He explained that he had recently been diagnosed with Alzheimer's disease. And, while he still had the cognitive ability, he wanted to spend more time with us if we were willing.

My immediate reaction was to get up and walk directly over to Mike and just hold him. Here was my dear friend—the jokester, the big kidder—announcing that he would soon lose his ability to think clearly. Impossible! These things happen to other people, but not to my friend, he's too young!

There were tears that day, as we talked openly of his fears and ours. We vowed that our visits would happen more frequently. We pledged we would spend our allotted time—time that had now been newly defined as finite—as well as we could.

I think we did, I hope we did. Over the next nine years we visited each other and watched Mike and Rosalys bravely navigate all phases of his disease. Always there was a warm heart and hand to hold when we sat together.

Love, Margaret

INSIGHTS

- Margaret's account reminds us that friends are also affected when Alzheimer's comes into a couple's lives. They, too, feel the loss of a relationship that now needs to change—not forgotten or gone, but forever changed.

- While you may hesitate to ask your friends to help you at a difficult time, be aware that most friends will actually see helping as a joy and a privilege. Over time you will all discover that sharing the difficult times together only deepens your friendship. (More on that in the next chapter.)

- It's true that some friends may seem reluctant or distant at first about continuing their friendship in the same way. Try not to take their reluctance personally. If you give them a little time to process the news and are willing to be patient and informative with them, chances are they will come back to your friendship, stronger than ever.

- Friends make it possible for you to safely voice your greatest fears and allow you to cry and laugh, and we all need to do both sometimes.

CHAPTER 14

LEARNING TO ACCEPT
SUPPORT FROM OTHERS

What I eventually learned was that
requesting or accepting help with
Alzheimer's is not a sign of weakness
or surrender, it can be an act
of love and strength.

MIKE AND I WERE NOT ACCUSTOMED to asking people for help or bothering others with our difficulties. In the past, whenever a problem arose, Mike and I had always turned to each other for help, and that's how we tried to deal with Alzheimer's too. Especially in the beginning we approached it as a two-person team and, in that way, we were able to remain fairly self-reliant for quite a while.

But Alzheimer's is a progressive disease. As Mike's health and abilities declined, we found that I had to do more and more for him—first, more each year and, eventually, more each month.

The simple truth is that caring for someone with Alzheimer's can never remain a one-person job. No matter how hard you might try, there comes a day when you can no longer care for your loved one by yourself. That doesn't mean that moving to a care facility is your only option; but if you choose to continue providing care in your home, it does mean turning to family and friends at some point for help.

What I eventually learned is that asking for help is not a sign of weakness or surrender, it can be an act of love and strength. I remained the primary caregiver for Mike throughout his illness, successfully managing his care in our own home. But it wouldn't have been possible without the help of family, friends, neighbors and, later, professionals.

YOU ARE NEVER ALONE

Being diagnosed with Alzheimer's can be a very lonely feeling but, as Mike and I learned, you are not alone—you are never alone. Your friends, family, neighbors and community are here for you too.

As time went on, I eventually had a small team of people helping me care for Mike. But I like to think of them not as a team but as a "circle" of thoughtful people who surrounded us and helped care for our physical, emotional, and spiritual needs.

The "help circle" started with our own adult children, Patrick and Kathleen, who were there for us from the beginning—first, by recognizing that something was wrong with Dad, and then stepping forward to help in every way they could. The really amazing part is that they never questioned our somewhat unorthodox choice of having Mike stay at home instead of in a care facility. They simply honored our choice and pitched in to help.

Then, one by one, along came our friends and neighbors who thoughtfully recognized that we had a need of one kind or another and offered to help, each in his or her own way.

When Mike was still healthy, he had pitched in to help his good friend Stan build a house for his wife, Audrey. Even with Alzheimer's Mike could hold a board or fetch a hammer for Stan, always encouraging coffee breaks, and bringing laughter to the project. Now that his friend Mike needed a little help with Alzheimer's, Stan was right there for him too. When Stan and Audrey heard that Mike could no longer be left alone, they offered to have Mike stay with them one day a week—amazing!

When I mentioned to my friend, Wendy, that I was going to have to quit our book club to keep Mike company, she and her husband Art offered to have Mike stay with Art on our book club nights. That meant that I could still have a night out with the ladies now and then—wonderful!

Then there were our next-door neighbors, Gary and Linda, who were always ready to give a helping hand. I hope they realize how comforting it was for me to know that they were there in case of an emergency. I didn't need help often, but their steady presence gave me so much confidence, or perhaps I should say courage.

For a long time, Mike and I managed pretty well with a little help from close friends and family. As I described earlier in Chapter 7, I was even able to continue working and teaching outside our home—all thanks to our circle of help.

THE CIRCLE GROWS

The first person we hired to help care for Mike was Stephanie, a family friend. Later we hired Sabina, a professional caregiver. Both of them became angels for Mike and me, especially during the last year of his life. (More about them in coming chapters.)

My sisters, too, became part of our circle, traveling from afar—Colorado, California, Nevada, and Alaska—and each finding her own special way to help.

When we finally asked, Father Dennis and the entire congregation from our church came forward with either prayers or a helping hand.

And there were others, too, such as Kirt the contractor who found a way to expand our bedroom by a needed three feet the year before Mike died. "I live just down the road," he assured me. "Call anytime if you need help with anything else, night or day." As it turned out, I did not need to take him up on that offer, but it was still a great gift to have his standing offer in my back pocket.

Another wonderful surprise came in the form of Marilyn and Claudia, our old friends from San Pedro. They came all the way from California to Bainbridge three times the last year to help with meals and whatever needed to be done. And they brought one of the best medicines of all—laughter—right when we needed it most.

And completing the circle were the professionals: Dr. Jung, Mike's doctor; Janelle, his physical therapist; Carol, his trainer; and, finally, the compassionate hospice team, including a registered nurse, a social worker, an aide, a Chaplin, and a massage therapist.

So why do I tell you these things? I tell you because I want you to remember that you have a circle too. You may not know it yet, but it is already building around you. Watch for it, welcome it, be thankful for it. Yes, it's a little scary at first to allow people in when you feel most vulnerable. But if you and your loved one do plan to stay in your home together, then you, too, must allow yourself to turn to a circle of caring people who can help you.

As the old saying goes, "You alone can do anything, but you can't do everything alone." If you reach out for help, I promise you that help will reach out for you.

INSIGHTS

- Telling people that Mike had this devastating disease was not easy. Later on, asking people for help was just as difficult, but we gradually realized it must be done.

- Once we learned to graciously accept the help that was offered, everything got a whole lot easier and better.

- For us there was an ongoing screening process. We asked ourselves: "Was this the right help from the right person at the right time?" If not, don't be afraid to decline an offer of help, even if it's from someone close to you.

- Some might call it a "team" but I like to think of it as a "circle" because it felt safe, interconnected, loving and never-ending.

- Each of the wonderful caring people in our circle gave a little of themselves on an emotional level too. Many had known Mike before and now they were witnessing the slow process of his decline. Alzheimer's takes a toll on anyone who participates in the care of someone with the disease. I hope that I was always kind and appreciative to the people who reached out to help Mike and me—they deserved it.

- So take care of your circle the best you can, catch your friends, family and neighbors doing something right and praise them for it. Remember, caregivers need care, too.

CHAPTER 15

THE ANGELS NEXT DOOR

*Alzheimer's makes us realize that
kindness and compassion are
reciprocal and near at hand.*

MY GRANDMOTHER LIVED HAPPILY ON HER OWN in a little apartment until age 97. That was only possible because of a good neighbor who watched for Grandma's curtains to be opened each morning. If the curtains were open, the neighbor knew my grandmother was okay; if they were closed, the neighbor knew they should walk over and check up on her.

That may seem like such a simple courtesy—and it was—but that little neighborly act of kindness made all the difference in the final years for a proudly independent woman.

Mike and I had similar acts of kindness bestowed on us by our next-door neighbors. Gary and Linda lived right up the hill at the end of our driveway. Over the years we had borrowed eggs, watered each other's lawns, and brought in each other's mail.

More importantly, Mike and I could tell that Gary and Linda were the kind of goodhearted people who would always be there for us if we ever needed them, and vice-versa. As it turned out, that comforting thought made all the difference in my ability to continue the quality of Mike's home care, especially in the mid and later stages of his illness. Here's just one example:

STUCK IN THE TUB

Mike and I had a Jacuzzi tub for two in our master bath. It was a favorite place for our little conversations and relaxing moments. If we had just wanted to be safe, we would have probably discontinued the Jacuzzi when Mike was first diagnosed. But, despite Alzheimer's, our relaxing soaks in the tub were one of those things we wanted to keep in our life for as long as possible.

One day, on a cool Sunday afternoon, Mike and I were in the mood for a nice warm Jacuzzi. Mike was in the eighth year of his illness, but still walking and physically strong. Helping Mike get into the tub was easy, and our chat that day was so pleasant that we probably lingered too long. When I tried to help Mike out of the tub, he did not have the strength or the ability to get up. Now what?

I tried emptying the tub, giving Mike chocolate covered coffee beans to perk him up, and finally decided to call our neighbors, Gary and Linda. I hated to bother them, but I didn't know where else to turn.

So here came Gary and Linda to the rescue. One quick call from me and down the driveway they came. With Mike looking sheepish in his boxer shorts, Gary climbed right in the tub, put his arms under Mike's and with a mighty lift pulled him up to a standing position. From there Linda and I could help lift Mike safely out of the Jacuzzi. Mission accomplished.

Now, I'm pretty sure that Gary and Linda will be astonished to see themselves portrayed as angels in this story. For them, it was no big deal to drop whatever they were doing and give their neighbors a helping hand. They made Mike and me feel like it was no problem at all that day, just a routine part of being a good neighbor.

So here is my message to Gary and Linda: You have no idea how often Mike and I were able to do something just because I knew you were there if we really needed you. Like my grandmother's neighbor, your comforting presence at the top of our driveway made all the difference for Mike and me in his final years. Thank you.

- Remember: On your journey with Alzheimer's, you are not alone. Your friends, family, caregivers and good-hearted neighbors are here too.

- Don't forget to exchange phone numbers with your neighbors, and post it by your phone. Chances are you may never need it, but if you do you'll be glad it's handy.

- Some neighbors may still shy away from those with Alzheimer's, for they have not yet learned it is not a disease to be feared. Be patient with them, for they too will soon learn from you and others just what this disease is all about.

- Through the years I learned to think of 9-1-1 as one of my neighbors. You don't want to call your neighbors or 9-1-1 unnecessarily; but you shouldn't hesitate to call either one when you're in need.

- Three times I called 9-1-1 to help when Mike had fallen and I couldn't get him up by myself. Each time the paramedics were big, strong, willing, and kind. They never made us feel like it was inconvenient for them. "This is what we are here for," they said.

- Alzheimer's helps us realize once again that kindness is reciprocal. If you want help now and then, be willing to help others. If you want great friends and neighbors, be one. That's how it works.

CHAPTER 16

A PRICELESS GIFT FROM
TWO OLD FRIENDS

Buck and Ellie gave Mike and me
a glimpse of the road ahead.

IF YOU ARE VERY LUCKY you will have people in your life who can give you a preview of what lies ahead. And sometimes these people are even willing to mentor you by sharing their experience and showing you what awaits around the next bend. Mike and I were lucky that way, for we had Buck and Ellie in our lives.

Buck and Ellie lived in a picturesque part of Montana fondly referred to as Mountain Brook, named after the babbling brook that runs alongside the dirt road. Mike's dad Peelo lived across the road from them in a little cabin he built. Buck and Ellie were originally good friends with Peelo and then became our friends too.

Buck worked for the Social Security Department and drove into town to work each day. He was a gardener, a wine maker, a donut baker, and a World War II vet, a member of the elite 101st Airborne Division who did their part on D Day, not to mention a great neighbor and friend.

Once a month, Peelo would catch a ride with Buck and go into town to buy his supplies. When Buck and Ellie's big garden overflowed with fresh fruits and vegetables each summer, Peelo reaped the rewards. Buck also had a full root cellar, which included many different varieties of Buck's delicious homemade fruit wines. Mike's dad had long ago given up the pleasure of even a drop of wine, as it had proven to be too much for him. But Mike enjoyed all of Buck's wines, especially the rhubarb.

Mike and I made annual visits to Mountain Brook when the children were young and enjoyed many wonderful meals, warm welcomes and always lots of laughter in Buck and Ellie's kitchen. One of my favorite memories is Buck's early morning deliveries of his homemade donuts after our long drives to the cabin.

BUCK AND ELLIE BECOME OUR MENTORS

After Mike's dad died, Mike and I became the keepers of his little cabin. And Buck and Ellie, 20 years our senior, became even closer friends and mentors to us.

As time passed, Buck was physically unable to do all that he had done in the past. The day came when it was time for our friends to make a move. They bought a home in town, close to the grocery store and medical clinic and even built elevated garden beds so they could keep gardening. Our annual visits continued at their new home.

Buck was aging and needed some help from Ellie, but they were managing just fine, until one day he had a small stroke. Now Buck's care was too much for Ellie so, with mixed emotions, Buck was moved into a nursing home.

Mike and I did not visit Buck at his new residence but heard from Ellie that it was expensive and she did not know how long they could afford it. Once again, Buck and Ellie were our mentors. Now they showed us how to deal wisely and courageously with the last chapters of life.

Ellie continued to be Buck's advocate and caregiver. She visited him daily, always watchful of his comfort and needs and their diminishing savings. Then one day on a phone call she told me she was moving Buck to the VA hospital. It would be a little farther away, 30 minutes or so, but he qualified, and the cost would be just half.

OUR LAST VISIT WITH BUCK

The VA hospital is where Mike and I had our final visit with Buck. At this point, Mike was about three years into his battle with Alzheimer's and was having difficulty expressing his thoughts.

When we visited Buck that day, we knew it was getting close to the end for him. Still, Buck looked calm and composed in his clean private room. He lay in a low bed which had been taken off the frame so he would not fall. This made him safe, but it was difficult for us to sit close to him. Ellie sat by his side, and Mike and I sat nearby as we had our final chat with our old friend Buck.

I don't know exactly what was said that day, I hope we told him how special he had been to us, and that we admired him, and we would miss him. I don't think we did, I think we said, we are glad to see you and it is a beautiful day out. I do remember Mike bending close to Buck and saying just the right thing, it might have been simply, "We love you."

Buck and Ellie had no way of knowing how important that visit was to Mike and me. Without realizing it, Buck and Ellie were showing us some of what lay ahead for Mike and me. We could no longer look away from the end of life, or avoid talking about it, because it was right there in front of us. Buck and Ellie were giving us a gift; they were showing us the end of life and helping us prepare together for where Mike would soon go.

After we left Buck's room that day, Mike began to talk. His words, at that point, were difficult to understand. But there was no doubt in my mind what he was telling me, as he bounced between talking about Buck and himself. Here is one of the notes I made in my journal that day:

⟶ FROM MY JOURNAL ↢

*Saw Buck at the VA hospital. It was sad but helpful. It prompted
conversation for us. As we walked to the car, Mike said,
"Buck still inside there somewhere."
Then, as we sat in the car, Mike went on to say, "Even when
don't think someone is there. Maybe they can't talk or tell you.
I think they still know."*

Mike was telling me that he believed Buck was still "there" even though he could not speak or show us in any way. Mike was also telling me that he believed he would still "know" what was happening as time went on and his illness progressed, even when he could no longer speak.

Mike went on to tell me the things that would be important to him at the end of life. They were simple but profound: He would want me to be with him, not to be a burden, for me to know that he would still be "there" and that he would "know" even when he could not speak or communicate. He wanted us to keep laughing, and he thought that it would be nice to have classical music in the room when he had come to the final days.

Here we were, two and a half years after Mike's diagnosis. For months Mike and I had been talking about durable power of attorney, his will, and staying at home with Alzheimer's, but we had completely missed what was most important about the last chapter of life. It took that final tender visit with Buck to prompt a conversation we should have probably had long before.

Buck and Ellie gave us a priceless gift that day. Even though the end of Mike's life was still years away, I now knew what Mike believed it would be like for him at the end of his life and what he would want for him and me during his last weeks.

Our visit with Buck that day often came to mind years later as Mike and I spent our last days together with classical music in our room, a hospital bed set up so I could sit close to him, laughter when I could, and always remembering: Mike was in there somewhere.

INSIGHTS

- Mike believed he would still "know" as he approached the end of life. That is the great question—how much does a person with Alzheimer's really "know" when they can no longer communicate and are at the end of life? I don't have the answer to that, but maybe Mike was right. Maybe it is more than we might think.

- Buck and Ellie gave us many gifts. Gifts come from all different places, the important ones are not always wrapped up neatly and tied with ribbon. They are just lying there in plain sight for us to accept if we are open and receptive to them.

- Perhaps Mike and I gave Buck a parting gift too. While I don't know that we said the right things our last day with Buck, maybe just being there at the end in that simple room in the VA hospital was our gift to him.

- Today, Ellie remains in their Montana home, continuing to garden and to be a mentor for me. For she has walked this path alone—as I do now—much longer than I.

- Whenever I visit Mountain Brook, Ellie and I enjoy a picnic lunch by the babbling brook, or a little day trip to our favorite place—Glacier National Park. We ride and talk of our old memories and of our husbands we still remember and love.

- Look around and you might be lucky enough to find a mentor or two to guide you along the way, or perhaps you will find that you can be a mentor for another Alzheimer's couple now or down the road. I hope that the thoughts in this book are being helpful to you and your loved one in that way too.

- Thank you, Buck and Ellie. What a difference you made for Mike and me.

PART V

~

Resolving Our
Differences

CHAPTER 17

ARGUMENTS WILL HAPPEN

*Halfway around the world,
Mike and I discovered that, despite
Alzheimer's, we could resolve a
passionate disagreement together.*

DURING OUR TRIP TO AUSTRALIA AND NEW ZEALAND, Mike and I found ourselves locking horns. It was our first significant argument since he had been diagnosed earlier that year, and I'm proud to say that both of us rose to the challenge to resolve it. Here's what happened:

We had enjoyed two wonderful weeks in Australia with our niece and were now on our own in New Zealand. The plan was to first rent a car and then, later, a camper. While signing the papers for the rental car at the Christchurch airport, I realized that Mike had every intention to drive.

Now, Mike and I had been doing pretty well with the driving issue. We still had no formal agreement between us, but I had stopped pressuring him to give up the keys. Accordingly, he had been cutting back on driving solo, and I had been taking the wheel whenever we were together.

But driving in a foreign country was not something we had talked about. I just assumed that I would drive, and he just assumed that he would drive. In Christchurch he quickly took the keys from the rental car agent and was not giving them up. I didn't argue, I simply suggested that perhaps I should drive. He said, "No, I will drive." And so he did.

MIKE & ME

Right after leaving the rental car lot, we found ourselves in a traffic circle and I knew we were in trouble. It took Mike forever to figure out how to get out of that circle, we just went around and around. But his driving seemed okay, and a traffic circle can be tricky for anyone, so I hung in there.

The next day we headed up a beautiful mountain pass with a green valley far below. It was a small, two-lane, twisty road with a stomach-churning drop-off on our left. As we traveled up the road, Mike kept drifting over the centerline, and then veering back toward the edge of the drop-off as we rounded the corners. The narrowness of the road and his speed were more than concerning, they were outright dangerous.

As I felt my shoulders tense, I attempted a calm reminder to Mike to slow down. Mike knew how to drive fast on winding roads and it was something he enjoyed doing. The problem was, he could no longer do it!

Despite my warnings, his speed did not decrease and he continued to swerve toward the cliff's edge. One more turn toward the edge and I reached over, grabbed the wheel and pulled us over to the other side. Mike was really mad, red-faced and silent. At the next pullout, he parked the car, got out, slammed the door, walked to the edge and just stood there. I feared he might step right over that cliff, and I began to cry.

Why did I ever think we could go to New Zealand? This was a mistake. What were we doing here, and what was I going to do now? The one thing I knew for sure was that Mike was not going to continue being the driver on this trip.

I also knew that talking to Mike or approaching him at that moment was the wrong thing to do. We both needed time to calm down. Here we were in the middle of nowhere, all by ourselves, and I had a husband with Alzheimer's whom I could not talk to or count on.

Mike stood out there for what seemed like a long time, and I just sat in the car with my tears and my fears. I didn't like it when we went our separate ways, I liked to talk things out together, but this was not one of those times. I was sorry for grabbing the wheel—and sad that Mike was upset—but I was not going to let him drive.

Eventually, Mike came back to the car, gave me the keys, and said, "You drive." He was still mad and his tone was not pleasant, but he said no more. I remained the driver for the rest of the trip.

Later, after we took the break you need after a fight, we calmly commiserated about the difficulty of driving on a different side of the road, and in a place you do not know. I hoped that conversation helped Mike maintain his position as the man, the one who liked to drive, the one who was the better driver, the one who had taken the driver's training program with the sheriff's department, the one who could drive backward through cones, and the one who had taught me to drive in the Montana snow.

I can only guess how difficult that moment must have been for Mike. Clearly, he was losing the battle with Alzheimer's. No matter how hard he tried, he simply could not do all that he had done in the past. Mike gave me no more angry looks and I stopped crying; we simply continued our trip with me at the wheel.

MIKE TO THE RESCUE

For our next adventure we returned the car and rented a camper, one of those big, high, fully-equipped vans. Let me tell you, they are just right for two to sleep and cook in, but I wasn't sure I could actually drive this thing. Nevertheless, the rental agent guided me through a brief practice drive in the lot and off we went.

Right away I entered the same roundabout again and, to Mike's delight, I ended up going around and around just as he had. We had a good laugh about that and then continued on.

Because the van was so tricky, it seemed best to head out to the country, away from city traffic. Once I got out of the roundabout, I drove down a country road to gain some confidence.

Okay, that went well, so I decided to try turning the van around. Simple, right? I would just make a turn in the middle of this country road and then put it in reverse. The problem was, I couldn't find reverse! There was no big "R" on the gearshift, and no manual in the glove box. Now what? I knew how to get into reverse in our VW camper—press down and up—no, that didn't work. Each time I made a new attempt, the van lurched a little closer to a country mailbox. *Yikes!*

I knew Mike probably couldn't help, but I so wished he was behind the wheel at that moment. More attempts, and more inching toward the mailbox. I was certain the cows in the nearby field were going to tell on me, and the farmer would arrive with pitchfork in hand. The attempts and inching seemed to go on forever!

Then, out of the blue, Mike said calmly, "Try pulling the gearshift nob straight out." I did and we were finally, blessedly, in reverse. Who would have thought—only Mike. He was my hero once again. When I asked how he knew this, he said it was like a tractor. Hmm, an experience I had not had, but one my dear husband had.

We returned to the open road, and continued our adventure in New Zealand. It could have easily turned into a disaster, but we had stuck together, remained patient and weathered the storm. Result: the good feelings and the mutual confidence were back in our relationship again.

INSIGHTS

- With Alzheimer's, arguments will happen as they do in all relationships. Don't fear them for they can be an opportunity for you to enter your partner's world and understand what he or she is feeling.

- In the middle of our fight, Mike and I took a break to cool off. That's a good tool for everyone, not just Alzheimer's couples.

- A good break is one where you can stop thinking about the stressful situation. I think that leaving the car and focusing on the quiet green valley below provided that for Mike.

- I was not angry at Mike during our break. I only had sad thoughts, about how things were changing, how it was harder now for us to go places, and about how difficult this must be for Mike, who was struggling with Alzheimer's.

- In an ideal world, we would have discussed things calmly after our break and listened to each other's perspective, and then perhaps compromised. But that was no longer possible because Mike's vocabulary was now more limited so it was becoming difficult for him to verbalize his feelings. Still, we got through it with love and patience.

- Because Mike couldn't express himself very well, it was up to me to guess out loud what he might be feeling, and then give him an opportunity to agree or disagree with what I said. After that, I called up good memories from our past days together. I praised him for being the better driver all our marriage and for helping me learn many things about driving through the years. And I sincerely assured him that I would need his valuable help in other ways (such as directions and signs) during the balance of our trip—but that I would be the one doing the driving.

- There could be no compromise about who would drive for the rest of the trip; I would be the driver. And yet I think Mike came away feeling valued by our talk.

- Keep having fun. Mike and I both agreed that if our argument was necessary for the trip to continue, then it was well worth it.

- Never forget that the person with Alzheimer's might know more than you think!

CHAPTER 18

THE BATTLE OF THE CAR KEYS

Here's what happened when I asked
Mike to give up driving for good.

OF ALL THE CHALLENGES WE ENCOUNTERED during the early years of Alzheimer's, Mike's determination to keep driving was probably the most contentious. Convincing someone you love to relinquish their car keys can be an emotional and complicated issue for both parties, and one that you'll likely encounter too, which is why I tell you this story.

Mike loved cars. He would point out vintage cars as we drove down the road, calling out the exact year and model, and then reciting the lore and legend of that particular vehicle.

When I first dated Mike, he drove a quirky 1954 English Ford. He really liked that car. It was missing the front passenger seat, so I sat in the back—oh well.

As a Federal agent, Mike learned how to drive fast and smart. He could zip expertly into small parking places that I wouldn't even consider. So, of course, in our daily life Mike was the "official driver" whenever there was ice or snow on the road, or whenever we were driving long distances.

After retirement, it was Mike who drove frequent errands to the grocery or hardware stores, took care of our car maintenance, drove to church for volunteer work, drove me to the ferry depot on the days I worked and picked me up at night when I returned.

Yes, Mike loved cars and he loved to drive. Then one day a doctor at the UW Medical Center suddenly asked him to give up his car keys. I had no idea, at first, how traumatic that request would be for him. What happened next was a lesson in love and patience for both of us.

—✦ FROM MY JOURNAL ✦—

APRIL

Today, Dr. S. at the University of Washington gave us the results of the Alzheimer's test and then told Mike not to drive. She said that the diagnosis would make us liable if he had an accident.

~

Friday, Mike and I talked. He is very angry over the no-driving issue. He told me his driving is fine and he is not going to stop. Furthermore, he feels this is his issue, not the doctor's or mine, and it is up to him to handle it.

I accepted what he said and explained that I would not take on the role of telling him not to drive. I would have to trust his judgment. He asked why I was concerned. I gave him multiple examples: Over the white line on the right side of the road on long-distance trips; 50% of the time no signal used; crossing lanes with no signal; almost hit the right side of the car when turning left (missed cars parked on curb by inches); and multiple fender benders.

~

Saturday, I told Mike how lonely it felt to be a "me" and not a "we". If he needed to do this (car thing) alone and it was all about him, then it means I need to do Alzheimer's alone too. I know I might eventually have to do Alzheimer's without him, but I don't want to have to do that now. He heard me and said, "We won't let that happen."

Looking back, I remember that weekend conversation like it was yesterday. It would have been easy to let the painful Friday night conversation sit and not be spoken of on Saturday, and yet I knew it was important to come back to the conversation the next day when we had calmed down.

Having calmed down, Mike was able to assure me that I would not have to do this Alzheimer's journey alone—and that was a great relief to me. The knot in my stomach went away. I knew that living with this disease would not be easy for us, but I also knew we could make it manageable as long as we traveled the road together.

HOW WILL WE EVER RESOLVE THE DRIVING ISSUE?

Of course, "traveling together" doesn't mean that you won't have disagreements; it means that you will try to understand and appreciate each other's point of view when you do disagree.

As it turned out, Mike and I were stuck on the driving issue for months. My view was that we at least needed to cut back on how much he drove. So I did all the driving when we were together, and Mike drove on his solitary trips around town. This decreased Mike's driving by about 70 percent, but neither of us was completely happy with that.

Mike remained angry at the doctor, and angry at me for siding with her. We rarely spoke about the driving issue and, when I did bring it up, he accused me of trying to "manage" him. I wondered how we would ever get "unstuck" on this issue.

The turning point came when we made a trip to Sacramento and had a visit with Mike's old college friend, Herb, and his wife. Having a third party that knew and loved both Mike and me allowed us to talk about the issue and not be judged. They listened while Mike and I both opened up about our conflicting perspectives on driving.

On the way home Mike and I discussed the driving issue in ways we had never done in the past. After months of being stuck, we both began to hear for the first time what the other person was actually thinking and feeling.

WE FINALLY UNDERSTOOD EACH OTHER'S POINT OF VIEW

As Mike and I continued to discuss driving, I began to appreciate how truly painful this issue was for him. Discovering that he had

Alzheimer's was tough enough to accept, but giving up his car keys was too much for him.

From Mike's perspective, if his driving was okay before he went into the doctor's office, then why was it suddenly not okay when he walked out? He had an issue with being declared a "bad driver" simply because he now had a diagnosis of Alzheimer's.

As we talked more I also began to understand how symbolic it was for him to give up driving. One minute he was a man, a husband, an expert driver—and the next minute he was losing his freedom, his independence, his power, his ability to take care of me, and yes—that includes driving to the store to buy a dozen eggs! That was the part I needed to better understand and appreciate.

And, for his part, Mike began to understand and appreciate my perspective too: that I actually felt sad about trying to limit his driving; that I didn't like this situation any better than he did; that it's no fun being the sole driver in a marriage; and that I was sincerely worried about our safety, and the safety of others.

Mike was still driving and I was still nervous and watchful, but at least we now understood each other's perspectives and were working together and communicating. From there, I reached out to the Alzheimer's community for more information on driving. What I discovered surprised me.

WAS MIKE RIGHT ABOUT DRIVING AFTER ALL?

One day I heard a doctor from the University of Washington Medical Center being interviewed on NPR Radio. She said that having Alzheimer's did not necessarily mean you could not drive. She explained that old motor skills such as riding a bike tend to stay with you. This made sense, but it was different from what Mike and I had originally been told. Was there now new information on this topic?

I decided to call *The Alzheimer's Helpline* for clarification. The person I talked to was wonderful. (I wish I had used the Helpline sooner!) She explained that having Alzheimer's did not necessarily mean Mike could not drive. Each individual is different. The key question was: how was Mike's driving record? The answer to that was: fine—no tickets, no accidents.

Then a breakthrough idea came: Looking to the future, the Helpline explained that it was important to keep assessing Mike's driving ability and that it was a good idea to have a third party—such as a trusted friend or relative—do the ongoing assessments.

Aha—a third party! Have someone else besides me alert Mike when he should no longer drive. Why didn't I think of that? If we could just find a trusted third party, I could let go of obsessing over Mike's driving and not "manage" him. I hoped I could do that.

OUR GOOD FRIEND STAN TO THE RESCUE

After thinking it through, I finally decided to meet with Mike's good friend Stan. To my relief, Stan agreed to be the "third party" to assess Mike's driving and alert him whenever it became time to no longer drive. I worried that Mike wouldn't accept Stan's offer, but he was fine with it. I think he was relieved that I would no longer feel the need to be the watchdog.

At long last we had reached a simple, human, reasonable compromise. Mike would hold onto his car keys for now, but we had a mutually agreeable plan for the future. We would all continue to monitor the quality of Mike's driving, with Stan serving as the final decision maker.

One day I followed behind Mike as he drove to church by himself. All was well! He stopped at each stop sign, looked both ways and observed the speed limit the whole way. I was so proud of him.

It dawned on me that when I am riding in the car with Mike, I may be talking and distracting him from his driving. My observation of his driving when I was not in the car helped me appreciate that he was still a safe driver, at least at this point in his illness.

A passage in my journal says that Mike stopped driving about two-and-a-half years after our initial doctor's appointment at the University of Washington Medical Center. And he stopped, just as we had agreed, when Stan and Dr. Jung said it was time.

Mike had been right! Having Alzheimer's did not necessarily mean he could no longer drive safely. The reality is that every person is different.

Looking back, I'm glad that we were able to work through this difficult situation reasonably and thoughtfully as a couple. That is my wish for you and your loved one too.

─────────────── **INSIGHTS** ───────────────

- Driving can be deeply symbolic for Alzheimer's patients—so be patient and empathetic. With Alzheimer's, empathy and patience can sometimes run out, but try to hold on for the next supply. It's worth it.

- Some individuals with Alzheimer's can drive safely for a time, and some cannot, so monitor your loved one's personal abilities and treat him/her as an individual.

- I was learning that my experience in teaching relationship skills for couples was continually valuable for me and Mike during our Alzheimer's journey. In this case: taking a break when Mike and I had a disagreement about driving; coming back to the topic when we were calm; appreciating the other person's perspective; and understanding that we both had to "yield" and give a little.

- I did not get everything I wanted nor did Mike. I got to drive whenever we were in the car together, and he got to keep driving when he was alone—sometimes. But the important thing is that we worked it out together as a couple.

- Your friends can help you when you need to discuss a touchy subject such as driving. Once Mike was willing to talk with both me and his friends, it became easier for us to talk about the subject together.

- The Alzheimer's Association and the 24/7 Helpline are there for you, with the latest information and support, not just on driving but on virtually any topic. I encourage you to reach out to them!

CHAPTER 19

AN ID BRACELET FOR MIKE?

Nope. He had no intention of
wearing anything that identified him
as an Alzheimer's patient.

AND NOW COMES A QUIRKY LITTLE SUCCESS STORY about my dear husband Mike and a clever invention he came up with. You will also learn how he and I found a good way to reach a compromise and cross another rocky road together.

Our story begins on the day Mike's physician, Dr. Jung, announced that it was time for him to consider wearing an identification bracelet.

Up until that day, Mike had gladly followed Dr. Jung's recommendations, and for good reasons. Each time we went to see our highly-regarded Seattle physician, she was prepared, gracious and caring. She carefully assessed Mike's skills, leveled with us about how things were progressing, and helped us remain positive about the next steps. Every Alzheimer's patient deserves the type of personalized treatment and care that Dr. Jung provided to Mike and me throughout his illness.

But then came the day when she announced it was time to start thinking about an ID bracelet for Mike. This occurred about two years after his diagnosis. As usual, Dr. Jung took the time to clearly explain her recommendation. She had a pamphlet that showed many different types of ID bracelets (they all looked fine to me) and she had valid points about why it was such a good idea to wear one, including:

- If Mike was lost and could not get home, then someone could check his ID bracelet and help him.
- His phone number would always be there on his wrist if he could not remember it.
- If he was ever in an accident and taken to the hospital, then they would know that he had Alzheimer's.

By the end of our visit with Dr. Jung I thought all this made perfect sense and was convinced that an ID bracelet was just the thing for Mike at this point in his care. We departed her office with the nice pamphlet and I felt quite certain that this would be an easy choice. Meanwhile, Mike said nothing.

IN NEED OF A COMPROMISE

Throughout our marriage Mike and I could usually resolve our differences simply by talking things through. Before Mike was diagnosed with Alzheimer's we had taken the Gottman Couples' Relationship workshop together. There we learned the wisdom of seeking a compromise, rather than a victory or defeat. Good thing, too, because the ID bracelet was about to become a big issue.

The day after we left Dr. Jung's office, I sat down with Mike to select an ID bracelet from the pamphlet—but I quickly realized that he was having none of it! He reminded me that he had never worn a bracelet of any kind, didn't like jewelry, and didn't even wear his wedding band. His trusty wristwatch was his only exception.

Nope. Mike had no intention of ever wearing an ID bracelet—that was for sure. And neither Dr. Jung nor I were going to change his mind on this one. What to do? I immediately fell back on some of the things I teach in the couples' relationship workshop and which Mike, too, had learned.

First, I suggested to Mike that we take a temporary break from this discussion. The break would allow us to avoid further conflict, hopefully making it easier for both of us to re-engage about ID bracelets later. And I vowed to myself that when we resumed the conversation I would do what Gottman calls a "soften start," which simply means starting the conversation more slowly and respectfully with your partner.

The break was good for both of us. The next time Mike and I talked we were both calm, but, despite my best efforts at a soften start, Mike was still determined not to wear an ID bracelet.

Hmm. This was not a fight like the one we had about driving in New Zealand, it was simply something we disagreed about and something we needed to figure out. Again, I thought about my couples' training and remembered something: maybe part of the problem was that we needed to better understand each other's perspective on this ID issue.

So I started there. Gently, I asked Mike to explain the reason for his refusing to wear a bracelet. Was it really his dislike of jewelry, or was there another reason? Slowly, he opened up to me. It turned out that his main reason was because he did not want to be identified as someone who had Alzheimer's.

Of course! Now I understood his perspective. As we continued to discuss the issue, Mike began to understand my main concern, too— that I was sincerely worried he might get lost and be unable to call me or get home.

MIKE'S GREAT IDEA

Now if we could just figure out how to compromise. For awhile we found a middle road that worked pretty well. We put a 3x5 card in his wallet with his name, our home phone, my cell, and our address. That was acceptable for both of us. Problem was, I knew this wasn't a long-term answer because Mike didn't always have his wallet with him.

A few weeks later Mike came up with an even better idea: he would have his name and phone number inscribed on his constant companion—his wristwatch. Great idea Mike. Off we went to a jeweler. Yes, they could add a little tag to the back of the band that would have his name and phone number on it. And they did just that.

Mike was so proud. He showed the new ID information on the back of his watch to his friend Stan, to our children and to anyone else who would listen. All the while I proudly recounted the story of how Mike himself had solved the identification bracelet problem, adding how clever and smart I thought he was to come up with such a creative idea, because he was.

The next time we went to see Dr. Jung, who had been following the ID discussion with interest, Mike very proudly showed her his clever watchband. She said, "What a great idea!"

Mike had won again, and I was glad!

INSIGHTS

- Like most good stories this one has a happy ending and a moral. The moral is: Just because someone has Alzheimer's doesn't mean that they are not smart and clever. So keep your loved one in the loop when choices are made, for they can often make a difference in their own care.

- Clearly, Mike's idea was not a perfect solution for me. Would Mike remember that the information was on his watchband? Possibly not. Would someone discover it on the back of his band? Well, I could only hope so!

- Perfect or not, however, his solution represented a successful compromise—and that was even more important. I didn't get it all my way and he didn't get it all his. This was something for me to remember. I wanted to continue being Mike's wife, friend and partner—not just a caregiver who always made him do what the doctor said, or what I wanted.

- Applying the couples' relationship information that I now taught at Swedish Medical Center helped me remember that there are always two different perspectives for every disagreement. This is true for all couples, not just Alzheimer's couples.

CHAPTER 20

UNDERSTANDING
ALZHEIMER'S ANGER

*Alzheimer's patients can reach
a point where they lash out in
frustration or anger at their
caregivers. If this happened as time
went on, I wondered how Mike and I
would survive that phase
of home care.*

IMAGINE IF YOU WERE DIAGNOSED with Alzheimer's. As the
years ticked by, you would feel your old personality and capabilities
slipping away.

First you would become sad about your plight, then frustrated,
then anxious, then fearful. Worse yet, as the disease progressed,
you would no longer be able to clearly communicate your feelings,
fears and frustrations to your friends and loved ones. No wonder so
many Alzheimer's patients eventually lapse into angry outbursts. If
you were in their shoes, you would probably feel that way too—we
all would.

But we are learning more about how to care for our loved ones.
In an effort to help caregivers cope with the different emotional
stages of the disease, the Alzheimer's Association continues to up-
date the latest research and recommendations. I have included one
of their helpful guides at the end of this chapter, but I urge you to
go to their site and read deeper. The more we all understand about
the causes of "Alzheimer's anger," the more we can lessen or prevent
it for our loved ones.

This chapter explains how Mike and I worked through his "anger stage." First I will tell you how Mike himself helped keep us out of that angry difficult place for a long time. Then I will share how our loving relationship and home environment helped us deal more effectively with the full-blown emotional meltdowns that so many caregivers have come to dread. In our case, Mike and I were able to come through that difficult period still safe, still in our home, and still very much in love.

HOW MIKE DIFFUSED HIS OWN ANGER

The unknowns were always the hardest part of Alzheimer's for me. Like everyone else, I had heard horror stories of how Alzheimer's patients could lose control and fly into a rage, especially in the latter stages of the disease. Not knowing when and if the disease would cause Mike to act that way is what made it so difficult. Would I be able to deal with Mike if/when he became angry and aggressive, and how long would we experience these scary emotions—days, weeks, or years?

It turned out that in Mike's case, it was not until the end of his ninth year that he started exhibiting some aggression and anger. Earlier—in the beginning and middle years—he did experience occasional anxiety and agitation, but here's how he himself was able to help us both cope with that:

Early in the disease Mike told me he had decided that he did not want to let himself become grouchy because of Alzheimer's, and he stuck with that commitment for years. In the occasional instances when he did become grumpy or difficult, I would call for a break and then, once he had cooled off, we would sit down together and talk about the problem. He would typically affirm again that he did not want to be like that and would give me a hug as his way of saying he was sorry.

This mutual respect and collaboration continued all the way into the ninth year of the disease and beyond. This suggests that, with the help of an informed caregiver, some Alzheimer's patients can maintain a semblance of control over anger and can make a conscious choice not to be grouchy. That's a gift Mike gave me, and perhaps your loved one can also help you more than you might think.

HOW LOVE AND FRIENDSHIP HELPED

As Mike's wife, friend and caregiver, I always tried to make our home environment easy and familiar for him. His toothbrush was always in the same place; the furniture was always positioned the same; the sounds and smells in our home were always familiar; and his care was always loving and consistent.

Through the entire course of the disease, Mike always knew that the people he loved were still there, he still had steady interaction with the world around him, and he still lived with the woman he loved. I believe that this helped him maintain his confidence, demeanor and composure.

As I mentioned elsewhere in the book, Mike and I maintained certain little rituals that helped us avoid anger and stay friends and in love, including:

- We kept our ritual of departures and reunions, with always a hug or kiss when I departed and when I returned.

- We had daily conversations. Even when Mike could no longer speak, I could tell him about my day, talk about his and help him verbalize his feelings.

- We knew that we should both seek to understand each other's feelings before trying to resolve our arguments or problems. (Mike did this longer than I ever expected.)

- We made sure to thank each other for little courtesies and niceties. Even at the very end of the disease Mike gave me a touch or looked me in the eyes as his way of expressing his gratitude.

- We took frequent breaks—naps for Mike and stepping away for me.

By maintaining a consistent environment and a positive, loving relationship, we managed to stay out of that angry aggressive place until the end of Mike's ninth year. By then he could no longer walk and could barely speak. The resulting frustration soon led to angry outbursts that could turn quickly into full-blown meltdowns, making me wonder once again: Can I continue to care for Mike in our home? Can I keep us safe and ensure that Mike doesn't fall or injure himself or me?

It turned out that I was not the only one who had to learn how to safely help Mike when he was having a meltdown. Here are two quick stories of how caring family members dealt with those episodes:

DAUGHTER KATHLEEN'S SCARE

One Sunday Kathleen, husband Sam and toddler Riley came to visit. They offered to go pick up takeout, but I said, "No I want to go, you stay with Dad," and, with that, I was out the door. (By this point in the journey I took advantage of every little break I could get!)

When I returned, I could tell something was wrong. Sam and Riley were downstairs, and Kathleen was attempting to calm her dad. It seemed that Riley had been listening to toddler music and playing with my childbirth education dolls that cry, and it was late in the day—a perfect set-up for Mike to have a meltdown.

I could see that Kathleen had responded perfectly: music off, dolls turned off, Sam and Riley sent downstairs, and Kathleen focused completely on calming her dad. At that point, I could step right in and it didn't take long for my familiar hug and reassuring words to calm Mike. Once Mike was calm, Sam and Riley returned from downstairs and we all moved on to a quiet family dinner. Disaster averted.

SISTER PATTY'S STORY

Here's how my sister Patty describes a difficult episode that she and her son Andy weathered with Mike:

"In January of Mike's tenth year I came down from Alaska to provide care for Mike while Rosalys taught a seminar. I was worried that this time I might not be able to care for him by myself so I asked my son, Andy, to join me.

"The day wore on and Mike was sitting calmly in his wheelchair. The next moment he became frustrated over something he was trying to communicate. As his frustration turned to anger, he became red in the face, tried standing up and reached out angrily at me with his arms. It was the only time I ever saw him in that aggressive state.

"When Mike finally collapsed back into the chair, he immediately looked sad, contrite, even ashamed. He hung his head, and his eyes filled with tears. His color returned to normal and his body seemed relaxed.

"I spoke softly to him and assured him it was okay. As I sat on the floor I rubbed the top of his foot and told him that I knew he loved me and would never hurt me. I told him how I knew it was just the disease that made him feel so bad and that I was sorry I could not fully understand, but no matter what we still loved each other and always would. He seemed to relax and understand.

"Although I was outwardly calm, inside I was a little scared. So when it was time to help Mike move from the chair I asked my son to help me. He came over, reached out his hand and asked Mike if he wanted to get out of the chair. Mike stared at him. Andy waited calmly, then repeated, 'Mike, do you want help?' Eventually Mike put his hand in Andy's and Andy was able to assist him out of the wheelchair and into the soft overstuffed chair."

SEEK FIRST TO UNDERSTAND

Often, as in Patty's story, Mike's outbursts stemmed from his frustrations and usually happened when I did not understand what he was trying to tell me. If I saw stress building, then I would attempt to divert his attention to a new activity or simply suggest to Mike, "Let's talk about this later." Sometimes it worked but occasionally it became a full-blown meltdown.

If I saw or heard that he was starting to escalate, I responded quickly. With Mike sitting I would approach from the side, put my arms around him, and give him a big loving hug. Immediately I would assure him that I loved him and then articulate the emotions that he could not verbalize himself: "Mike, I know this is really hard right now... it has been a long day... you worked so hard at moving in and out of the shower... you're doing such a good job."

At those moments I had to remember to FIRST understand Mike's honest feelings and not disregard them just because he had Alzheimer's or because I feared them. After I understood what Mike was trying to tell me, I then moved on to tell him what we could do to make it better.

As I hugged and talked to him, he would soon calm and, when it was time, I would tell him how I intended to help him: "Mike, I love you... you are at home with me... I am going to help you... you will be okay... you are tired, I will help you lie down."

ADDRESSING MY OWN FEARS

It is not surprising that when Mike's outbursts first started, my heart would race and fear would begin to build. What if Mike did not calm down, what would I do? However, it turned out that giving Mike a hug and talking calmly to him not only soothed him, it also soothed me. My own calming words reminded me that this was just a moment in time, a moment when the disease had taken over, and therefore a moment when I could help Mike like no other. I now knew even the most difficult moments would soon pass.

Of course, when Mike had a meltdown, I always had the option of giving him medication under his tongue to help him relax. But I did not want him to spend his last months in a medically induced haze. So first I tried hugging, listening and understanding, which usually eliminated the need for medication.

Finally, it was important for me to remember that Mike's meltdowns were scary times for him, too, because he had virtually no control over those unwanted feelings that came on so unexpectedly.

Again, Mike's safety (and mine) were always my highest concern. I knew Mike never wanted to harm me, but I did have to stay clear of his waving arms at the moments he had a meltdown. At this point in the illness, Mike was no longer walking so it was easy to come from the side and use my whole upper body to hug him. It worked perfectly and made me think of how you swaddle a baby to help calm them.

So Mike stayed safe and so did I, which meant we were able to stay in our home together a little longer. While I continued to wonder, "Can we do this until the very end?" I knew we were still okay for now.

It was love that helped me learn not to fear Mike's outbursts or meltdowns. With love I was able to understand him and to stay connected to him to the very end. My sincere hope for you is that by sharing our story you, too, will learn not to fear the angry emotions that Alzheimer's sometimes brings.

⤳ FROM MY JOURNAL ⤶
AUGUST (YEAR 9)

Anxiety starts in the evening, sometimes when Mike is explaining something that I cannot understand, and then escalates. If necessary, pills relax and calm Mike in about 20 minutes. It also makes the transfer to bed easier.

SEPTEMBER (YEAR 9)

Mike was angry and tearful last night, but today I gave him coffee, did exercise with him, got him heading to bed by 7:15, and read to him. I think all helped, no anger tonight.

OCTOBER (YEAR 9)

There are so many changes. Mike has been tearful and angry at times while I have been gone. Sabina (our caregiver) even called hospice for advice.

*Mike was upset and crying while sitting in the wheelchair looking
out our bedroom window. Power was out and we were eating
dinner in our room—still a little light but candles lit. I sat on the
bed and began to talk to him:*

Mike, you have Alzheimer's.

Sometimes things get confused.

It sometimes makes you angry or sad.

But, I love you

And you love me.

You've had Alzheimer's ten years and it's now getting hard.

We don't know if you will get better.

But, we have a plan.

I will take care of you.

You will stay at home with me.

We did nice things knowing this would get hard later.

Trips to Australia, New Zealand, Ireland, Hawaii.

*Now is the hard time, but we still have good times, too,
and continue to love each other.*

~

*Whenever I give Mike my little talk he calms. He even nods at
times when I ask if he understands. I sometimes tap our wedding
rings together and remind him we are married and go together.
It is amazing that he can still be connected in this way and
understands, or at least is able to calm with information.*

MARCH (YEAR 10)

*No more tears, now. Some yelling but it no longer scares me.
He settles so easy when I change activity.*

UNDERSTANDING A LOVED ONE'S
ANGRY OUTBURSTS

You can find detailed information about dealing with the emotional changes that might occur with Alzheimer's on the Alzheimer's Association web page (www.alz.org). For starters, here are some very useful tips the Association recommends to address and mitigate angry or aggressive behavior:

1. **Try to identify the immediate cause.** What happened right before the reaction that may have triggered the behavior?

2. **Rule out pain as a source of stress.** Pain can cause a person with dementia to act aggressively.

3. **Focus on feelings, not facts.** Rather than focusing on specific details, consider the person's emotions. Look for the feelings behind the words or actions.

4. **Don't get upset.** Be reassuring. Speak slowly in a soft tone.

5. **Limit distractions.** Examine the person's surroundings, and adapt them to avoid similar situations.

6. **Try a relaxing activity.** Use music, massage or exercise to help soothe the person.

7. **Shift the focus to another activity.** The immediate situation or activity may have unintentionally caused the aggressive response. Try something different.

8. **Decrease level of danger.** Assess the level of danger—for yourself and the person with Alzheimer's. You can often avoid harm by simply stepping back and standing away from the person. (If the person is headed out of the house and onto the street, be more assertive.)

9. **Avoid using restraint or force.** Unless the situation is serious, avoid physically restraining the person. He or she may become more frustrated and cause personal harm.

10. **Share your experience with others.** Join ALZConnected, the Alzheimer's Association online support community.

─────────────── **INSIGHTS** ───────────────

- Whenever Mike had a meltdown, I saw it as an opportunity for closeness and tried to understand his feelings first and then and only then help him resolve the problem.

- Mike's emotions at times were much like a young child's when they cannot make you understand what they are trying to tell you. I had to always remember how difficult it was for Mike not being able to get me to understand him.

- The Alzheimer's Association reminds us that the caregiver can make a difference in the number and intensity of unwanted emotions. I am convinced that Mike's home environment and his relationship with me did, in fact, make a huge difference in minimizing aggression and anger.

- At first it seemed that I could do so little to help him when he was stressed, but it turned out that my love and patience did much more then I expected. I could not stop the disease, but I could always pull him back to being Mike with patient loving words and touch in the most difficult moments.

- There were times when Mike's anger made it seem as if Mike was no longer Mike, but that was not true. Throughout the entire 10-year illness, Mike was always Mike. I just had to find ways to tap into who he was and not lose him in those brief angry moments when he seemed to no longer be with me.

CHAPTER 21

A WORD ABOUT YELLING

*There came a phase when—out of
the blue—Mike began yelling. This
new behavior wore me down and put
our mutual commitment to
home care at risk.*

NO MATTER HOW COMMITTED you are to caring for your loved one at home, there may be certain periods on the journey when you'll feel like you've come to the end of your rope. At those times you'll wonder, "Can I honestly continue to do this?"

One of those periods began for me in the winter of Mike's last year of life. It was then that he began to do something that was extremely demanding of me. Namely, my dear husband Mike began yelling whenever I was out of his sight—not just now and then, but virtually all the time. Suddenly, I could not leave the room to prepare a meal, or answer the door, or get his medication, or for any reason at all without him yelling in a loud distressed voice.

This new behavior of Mike's continued for days, which turned into weeks, which turned into months. It was exhausting; I began to lose my patience; and I admit that I began to think seriously about throwing in the towel on home care.

Nevertheless, I was committed to keeping the deal that Mike and I had made when he was first diagnosed. We had agreed that we would manage Alzheimer's together at home for as long as it was safe for both of us. Despite Mike's yelling, we were still safe and we were still managing home care, so I wanted to hang in there. The problem was that I was frustrated and exhausted by Mike's continual yelling. I knew I had to figure out how to negotiate this new bump in the road—and I finally did. Here's how I thought it through.

WHAT DIDN'T WORK

At first I thought Mike and I could somehow work this out together, just as we had worked through so many other problems in the past. So I tried getting Mike's help by gently explaining to him that he did not need to yell when I left the room because "I will be right back." However, at this point in the illness he either could not remember what I said or fully understand what I meant.

I then tried every creative idea I could think of, including a baby monitor so he could hear my voice from the kitchen; a recording of my voice; calming music; calling to him from the other room; and talking loud so he knew I was near. None of it worked.

WHAT DID WORK

One day I was returning home after teaching a class on newborn baby behavior and a thought came to me. As the ferry glided smoothly through the water I began to think about what this difficult period of the disease must be like for Mike and how it was similar to what happens with mothers and their babies.

There comes a time when infants cry whenever their mother is out of sight. We often say that the baby is being "fussy," but it's really a sign that the baby is becoming more and more attached to the mother. Still, as the crying continues, even the most loving and patient mother may feel frustrated, exhausted or even angry because her baby is constantly yelling for her. Could it be that something like this was happening with Mike and me?

Suddenly it all made sense. Even though it felt at times like Mike was yelling "at" me, I needed to remember that he was actually yelling "for" me. Despite the severity of this latter phase of Alzheimer's, he still felt closely connected to me and loved me. But, like a newborn baby, he no longer had the ability to know that I was nearby when I was out of sight—so, of course, he yelled for me.

Instead of dwelling on my own frustration, I now saw with fresh eyes just what this phase of the disease must be like for my husband Mike. And this made a huge difference in my ability to respond to Mike with greater empathy, love and patience.

By reminding myself to see things from Mike's perspective, I became a stronger, wiser, more capable partner when my husband needed me the most. This change in perspective is a tool that you can call on, too, not just in the difficult later stages of Alzheimer's, but all throughout the journey.

REMIND YOURSELF, "THIS WILL NOT LAST FOREVER"

Here's another "point of view" that helped me cope with the most difficult stages of Alzheimer's: when things in your life are weighing you down, remind yourself that nothing lasts forever, not even your problems. Every mountain has a top, and every problem has an endpoint—even with Alzheimer's.

I liken this to a woman in labor. When she comes to the most difficult and painful part, she thinks she cannot do it. But if she learns that she only has a short time until she enters the delivery phase, she regains the ability to hang on and make it through the pain.

That's how it was for me when Mike was in his "yelling phase." Just when I was starting to feel "I cannot bear this forever," a social worker from hospice told me that this phase wouldn't last much longer and soon we would enter a quieter time. That perspective made all the difference for me.

I'M GLAD I WAS PATIENT

The social worker was right, of course. Mike's yelling only lasted a little longer and then we entered a quieter phase that ultimately led to Mike's final days with me and our family.

Ironically, when Mike no longer yelled I missed his "calls" because those had essentially been some of his last words. He now slept more and was peaceful, but our house was too quiet and seemed less alive.

Mike was, however, still aware and had moments when he continued to tell me that he loved me by responding to my voice or being glad when I returned from work. He could no longer tell me that he loved me or missed me with his words or his yells, but he told me with his eyes and his touch. Even in the final days of his illness he would look me right in the eyes, would raise a hand to touch mine, and pucker his lips for a kiss. Those last tender "I love yous" will linger forever.

I hope I was patient enough with Mike during his most difficult times. I think I was.

INSIGHTS

- The term "object permanence" is used to describe a child's ability (or inability) to know that objects or people continue to exist even though they can no longer be seen or heard. In the last stage of Alzheimer's, Mike did not have that ability. Knowing this made it easier for me to understand his demanding behavior.

- People with Alzheimer's often behave differently from one another, so not everyone will go through a yelling period as we did. It is interesting to note, however, that yelling sometimes happens in care facilities when an Alzheimer's patient becomes attached to a caregiver.

- It is also worth noting that a three-month-old child understands your tone of voice, but not your words. A twelve-month-old child understands both your tone and your words. This gives us all hope that even those in the advanced stages of Alzheimer's may understand more than we might think.

- With Alzheimer's, not knowing how long a difficult time will last is especially difficult for the caregiver. Learning that some things would eventually get easier and not harder was a huge help for me.

- It's easy for a mother to become angry with a crying baby. It's easy, too, for a caregiver to become angry with a yelling partner and feel overwhelmed by the continual demands of the one they love. Here are some things you can do when you feel exhausted or frustrated:

  √ You can step away and take a moment to calm yourself. A few deep breaths can make a huge difference in how you handle a difficult situation.

√ If friends or family are available, you can ask for help.

√ If you are alone, explain to your loved one that "we" are having a difficult time right now, but "we" will figure this out.

√ Add extra help so you can take time away from your loved one now and then.

√ If necessary, have someone spend the night with you in your home so you can get some sleep.

√ Remind yourself this is only a limited period of time and will eventually pass.

- Both babies and Alzheimer's patients can test our patience, so it's up to us as caregivers to remain centered and loving in our response to them. By stepping away when I needed to, bringing in more help, and taking time away, I was able to continue to speak kindly and to give loving care to Mike who deserved no less.

CHAPTER 22

WHEN IS IT OKAY TO LIE TO YOUR LOVED ONE?

There will be times when a
well-intentioned lie will seem like
the easier road to take…
but, should you?

As a loving partner to someone with alzheimer's there will come a point where lying to your partner may seem much easier and more humane than upsetting them with the truth.

I remember when that day came for Mike and me. It was in the summer of the eighth year of Mike's illness. It started off as a happy day because he and I were headed to our favorite place—our cabin at Mountain Brook—for a much-needed getaway.

As we drove along on a quiet country road with a few pine trees scattered here and there, Mike said that he was looking forward to seeing his dad at the cabin. This was a problem, for his father had died some thirty plus years before.

Without realizing the devastating effect my answer would bring, I simply responded with the truth: "Mike, your dad died a long time ago." From there I started to fill in the details of what had happened, but Mike was already overcome with tears.

As his crying escalated, I pulled over under a shady pine. My shoulders tensed as I felt his mounting sadness and bewilderment. Clearly Mike was feeling the pain as if he was hearing of his dad's death for the first time. There we sat, all alone in the car on that hot summer day with Mike crying and me feeling anguish over telling my husband the truth.

I didn't know what to do next, so I just began to talk about the sad feelings Mike was having. I talked about Mike's dad and how sad it was not having him with us anymore; how he had given us the great gift of Mountain Brook; how we both missed him and loved him.

Mike's sobs were so great that I feared he would never break out of this sad place. But as I continued to acknowledge his feelings and talked lovingly of his dad, he began to calm.

From there, I spoke of how I was looking forward to seeing our little cabin again and listening to the familiar sounds of Mountain Brook, and what a nice time we would have. Slowly Mike came out of his deep sadness. We ended with a hug and then continued down the winding road that carried us to our beloved cabin.

HAD I DONE THE RIGHT THING?

We often hear that the truth hurts. Well, Mike and I had just experienced that pain firsthand. As we continued our drive that day, things became quiet, with each of us in our own thoughts. I wondered if I had done the right thing. Or should I have told Mike that his dad was away on a trip and would not be at the cabin when we arrived? I had miles to contemplate as Mike looked out the window and then slipped into a peaceful sleep.

What was done was done. I had caused Mike a great deal of grief and I did not want that to happen again. So what should I do in the future?

If I lied, then I would need to form a conspiracy with other liars. I would have to explain to friends and family that Mike doesn't understand and gets very upset if he hears his dad is dead—so don't set him off. I would have to remind our son and daughter, for example, "Don't talk to your dad about your grandfather, he thinks he is still alive."

If I lied to Mike about who was alive and who was not, then what about other lies? Would I lie when Mike didn't want me to go to work? Would I say I am just going to the store and would be right back when, in fact, I planned to be gone all day?

No, that kind of "humane lying" wasn't humane at all; in my eyes, it was more of a betrayal. After all, I knew Mike counted on me to help him keep things straight. Whenever he was confused I helped him get centered. I reminded him which way to go in the house, the actual time of day, the real day of the week, exactly where we were going that day, and what we were going to do. So why would I not help him with the big issues too?

No, I would not start lying to Mike; instead I would continue to help him keep things straight. But perhaps there could be an easier way than what had just happened, and here's what I finally decided:

Should the question of his dad come up again, I would be truthful, but not go into much detail. "Your dad is no longer with us," I would say. "He died, but we are lucky to have such good memories of him. We are so lucky to have Mountain Brook. The brook should be full and the leaves lovely at this time of year." If Mike asked for more detail I would tell him; otherwise, I would quickly move on to talk about more positive memories.

I now had the semblance of an ongoing "process" whereby Mike and I could continue to understand and deal with truth and every-day realities.

- I did not lie to Mike before and would not lie to him now.
- I would not play into his misconceptions, even for short-term convenience or to spare his feelings.
- When he was confused, I would tell him the truth.
- When the truth brought him sadness, I would listen and understand his feelings and then help him express them.
- From there, I would help him move to more positive thoughts or activities.
- I would not argue with Mike about what was true.
- If we disagreed, then I would simply say, I guess we disagree.

The question of who was alive came up again one day. While we looked at our wedding album Mike spoke of his mother as if she were alive—and I immediately turned to our process for help. I said gently but firmly to Mike, "Your mom died." And then I turned the page.

While I did not want to disregard his sadness, I did not want to trigger more sad memories either. So we moved on to talk about other happy memories on that wedding day, and in the end Mike seemed content with the photos and the stories they told.

Throughout Mike's illness, I continued to help him with his memory, always setting the record straight and telling him what was true. For the most part he seemed to get what I was doing, and did not go back to the confusion that was previously there on the subject. He simply needed a little help grappling with reality now and then.

So now you know what we did and why I think I made the right choice for Mike and for me. Now you get to decide what the right choice is for you and the one you love.

INSIGHTS

- There were times when a little lie seemed like the easy answer, but it was not the right answer for Mike and me.

- We chose to hold on to the truth through the entire illness, and I believe it helped Mike remain connected with me, his family, his friends, and the world around us.

- Even late in the disease, Mike's feelings were still real and were not to be disregarded.

PART VI

~

Learning to Compensate
and Keep Going

CHAPTER 23

KEEPING MIKE SAFELY
ON HIS FEET

*As Alzheimer's progressed, Mike's
ability to walk was decreasing while
the risk of a fall was increasing.*

NOW THAT SHE'S CONSIDERED TO BE "ELDERLY," my friend Ellie tells me that people keep warning her, "Just don't fall." She laughs and says, "I always want to tell them: Who wants to fall?"

Near the middle of the fifth year, when Mike first began to have problems with mobility, I, too began hearing, "Just don't let him fall." Falls are a real concern for people with Alzheimer's because a fall might cause a serious break...which might precipitate a stay in the hospital . . . which might deteriorate into a move to a nursing home...which might lead to becoming wheelchair bound or even bedridden.

As Alzheimer's progressed, Mike's ability to walk was decreasing and the risk of a fall increasing. The obvious fix, of course, was to simply throw in the towel and start using a wheelchair to get around. A wheelchair might be safer, but Mike and I were both committed to keep him walking. We were determined to keep things as normal as possible for as long as possible. And walking was an important part of keeping our lives normal.

Looking back, I can see now that we were quite successful. It took both of us working together, but we were actually able to keep Mike walking and standing even into the ninth and final year of our Alzheimer's journey. Here's how we approached it, and what we learned.

START WITH PREVENTION

Mike first began having difficulty with his footing about five years after he was diagnosed.

Our response at that early point was to simply do all we could to avoid the causes of potential falls. We made our home safer by removing throw rugs and other obvious tripping hazards. Later, I was constantly vigilant for problem areas such as steps, uneven surfaces, slippery places, or poor lighting. And Mike and I made it a rule not to rush him, so he could focus on maintaining his footing.

This was especially important when we ventured outdoors where curbs, ramps or steps presented a constant challenge. After a few early mishaps and falls, I decided I had to be by Mike's side whenever he went up or down a curb.

We learned that when Mike approached a curb or step, he had to slow his pace because he could no longer gauge exactly when to step up or down. Coping with curbs and steps created a little tension on our outings, but we learned how to navigate them together and continued on with life.

THE RIGHT ATTITUDE HELPS

No matter how careful we were, there were still occasional falls, but Mike and I basically adopted the attitude, "You just get back up, dust yourself off and keep going."

We decided not to be embarrassed by public falls. We just looked at them as little accidents or obstacles that we would take in stride for the sake of continuing a normal life together.

At first when Mike would fall he could get up by himself or with a little help from me. After a fall, I would give him a minute to be sure he was okay. Then, with an arm under his elbow, I would help him up. As the disease progressed, I would move a chair or bench to where he had fallen. As he pushed down on the chair I pulled up on his wide jean belt to give him a little extra boost until he was back on his feet.

Through all the frustrations, Mike carried on with courage and resolve. I remember a few times seeing tears in his eyes after a fall, but not from being hurt. I think it was just sadness for all that he was losing, or from seeing all that I had to do to help. I hope I did not say or do anything that made those moments of sadness more difficult for him. I wanted him to know how proud I was of him. I remember commenting in my journal that "Mike falls well and heals rapidly."

A good example was the day we decided to take the ferry to Seattle for some shopping and a visit to the art museum. As we walked toward the ferry, Mike tripped on a curb and fell. He avoided hitting his head, but his knee was scraped and bleeding.

We boarded the ferry anyway and the purser supplied me with everything I needed to patch a skinned knee. By the time the ferry docked in Seattle, Mike's knee had stopped bleeding but I wondered, "Should we turn around and go back home on the ferry, or continue on with our outing?" True to form, Mike wanted to continue on, so off we went with my arm under his elbow as we walked.

You may wonder if it was risky or foolish to continue with our outing that day, but it turned out that we made the right decision. Mike and I saw wonderful works of art, looked at beautiful purses, had a delightful lunch at a little French bakery, and even returned to buy a purse that Mike wanted me to have. Today I still carry fond memories of a day in the city with the man I loved.

WHY MIKE AND I JOINED A GYM

It's interesting to note that, when Mike was diagnosed with Alzheimer's, we asked about exercise and were told it would not make much of a difference. That advice is now changing. Today, the Alzheimer's Association recommends regular walking and other physical activity as a way to keep both the body and the brain as healthy as possible for as long as possible.

As Mike's struggles with balance and agility increased, we asked our doctor if physical therapy would help with his mobility. She thought it might, so off we went to physical therapy once a week.

Going to physical therapy turned out to be wonderful in three ways: Mike liked the therapist, who made him feel like he was doing a good job; we both enjoyed the outing together; and there was the added benefit that I was learning in therapy how to avoid hurting myself while helping Mike.

Jeanine, the physical therapist, taught Mike some stretching exercises and encouraged him to do them three times a week at home with me. This added to my "to do" list but it also created another positive activity for Mike and me to do together.

Next, my daughter and son suggested that perhaps a professional trainer might also be useful, someone to help Dad keep doing the exercises. So we went to the local gym with the physical therapy instructions in hand. It felt good to be taking another positive action together. This Alzheimer's was not going to beat us!

It turned out that Mike looked forward to going to the gym each Thursday, and so did I. It was like the old days, before Alzheimer's, when we use to do things like this together—so normal.

While Mike did his routine I would walk to the nearby Blackbird Bakery and enjoy a rare quiet moment and a cup of tea. Nothing could have been better.

THREE MOBILITY TOOLS FOR THE CAREGIVER

If your partner has Alzheimer's, let me urge you again to keep him/her as active as possible for as long as possible—not only for their own health and happiness but for yours as well.

As Mike's everyday caregiver, I didn't realize at first that caring for him would become much more difficult when he could no longer help by walking or standing. To put it another way, every day that Mike could walk or stand on his own was making our lives fuller and my job as caretaker safer and easier.

Over time we turned to three very helpful pieces of equipment to keep Mike on his feet:

1. The Gate Belt. Soon after we started physical therapy we purchased a Gate Belt at the therapist's office. It's a wide belt that fits around a person's waist and gives the caregiver a way to hold on to the person walking. This enables the caregiver to stabilize the person should they start to fall. By holding on to the Gate Belt, I was usually able to save Mike from falling. And if he did fall, then I could use the Gate Belt to help pull him back up. It also made me feel less edgy when Mike wanted to move around the house because now I always walked with my hand on the belt wherever he went. Credit Mike's positive attitude again, for he patiently put up with the Gate Belt and with me.

2. A Wheelchair. For years Mike and I resisted the idea of permanently surrendering to a wheelchair, but we did use one here and there to supplement his walking. As time passed, we relied on the wheelchair to get Mike to and from the car or to roll longer distances. Thanks to the wheelchair and close parking we were able to keep going to the gym safely for quite a long time.

3. The Sit-to-Stand Machine. There came a time when Mike couldn't stand, get out of bed or walk by himself, at least not predictably. At that point our caregiver Sabina introduced us to an amazing little invention called the Sit-to-Stand machine. By using this clever battery-operated "hoist," a solitary caregiver like me can pull their loved one easily and safely off a bed or chair and right up to their feet. The Sit-to-Stand machine made a huge difference in Mike's quality of life in the final year (see Chapter 44).

LIFE SLOWS DOWN, BUT MIKE AND I CARRY ON

With all these little tricks and techniques (plus a lot of determination and teamwork) Mike and I were able to keep him mobile or semi-mobile all the way into his last months. From there, things really slowed down. And yet, even when he could no longer walk, we still found ways to enjoy our time together each day.

When Mike could no longer walk, we continued our dates and outings by going to interesting places where Mike could stay in the car. For example, we liked to go to Rolling Bay, where Mike would wait in the car while I got his favorite coffee drink. Then we would drive to Fay Bainbridge Park to sip our drinks, and enjoy some fresh pastry or a picnic lunch in the car as we watched the waves. Sometimes we would see a huge ship sailing out from Seattle to begin its voyage across the Pacific and wonder what adventure was about to unfold for those on board.

As I review my journal from this period, I'm reminded that Mike's falls began to happen in the last two years of the disease. When a person who has Alzheimer's starts to have frequent falls, that's usually a sure sign the disease is progressing. Ultimately this leads to the inability to walk, or even stand, both of which place a bigger burden on the caregiver. Sadly, for some couples, this means they can no longer provide safe care at home for their loved one.

As you can see from our story, however, we found that regular exercise, physical therapy and stretching kept Mike on his feet long after many Alzheimer's patients have resigned themselves to a wheelchair.

Then, even when Mike could no longer walk, we found ways to have him stay at home with the aid of the Sit-to-Stand machine and, of course, the help of friends and family who were always there when we needed them most.

Figuring out how to keep Mike living in the home that we both loved when he could no longer walk was a big hurdle, but together we accomplished it. I hope that you can too!

INSIGHTS

- If you or your loved one has Alzheimer's, stay as physically active as long as you can. Resist the temptation to resort to a wheelchair or bed for as long as possible.

- Keep a positive attitude. Despite Alzheimer's, Mike and I were able to enjoy many years together. Try not to dwell on what you have lost; focus instead on what you have left.

- Mike's physical therapist and also Carol (a trainer at the gym) were incredibly helpful; we should have sought them out sooner!

- Helpful tip: We gradually decreased Mike's physical therapy visits and increased his time at the gym. The therapist had taught us all that we needed to know, and Carol could help Mike do the exercises at the gym, which was less expensive than continuing therapy.

- The simple stretching exercises that Jeanine designed felt good to Mike. (Example: Hold both ends of a closed umbrella and stretch your arms above your head.) I believe that stretching kept him limber longer than might have been the case otherwise.

- Whenever Mike fell, I did not tell him that he caused the fall, or scold him for being careless; we simply moved on and solved the problem together.

- Even as our life together slowed down, there were benefits for Mike and me in this new simplicity: No schedules to meet, no trips to make, just quiet times together in our home, or at little scenic places where we could drive and sit in the car, share the moment, and watch the world go by.

CHAPTER 24

WHEN WORDS BEGIN TO FAIL

*Mike's diminishing vocabulary
was a huge loss, but he and I found
other ways to communicate, long
after words had deserted us.*

ONE DAY, DURING THE MIDDLE YEARS of our Alzheimer's journey, Mike turned to me and asked, "What do you like and what do you don't like?"

After I answered those questions, I asked him in return, "What do *you* like and not like?" He answered sadly, "I don't like losing my words." (Did I put my arms around him then? I can't remember, but I hope so.)

When Mike was first diagnosed with Alzheimer's, we were cautioned to expect problems with memory and mobility, but no one told us how discouraging it would be to gradually lose (as Mike would say) "my words."

There is little written about people with Alzheimer's losing their ability to speak, and even less about how couples, friends and family handle this great loss as it progresses. Perhaps this is because it is too painful for any of us to ponder what it must be like to have the ability to speak taken from you.

The gradual decline of Mike's vocabulary (and how we handled the situation) is what this chapter is all about. As you will see, Mike's diminishing vocabulary was a huge loss, and yet he and I found other ways to communicate, long after words had deserted us.

Communication is so much more than words; it can be a look, a gesture, a touch, a troubled frown, or a faint smile. These and other subtle ways of communicating remained for Mike and me when words failed. For now, I will tell you about Mike's words, but in chapters to follow I will tell you more about the many ways Mike stayed connected and communicated with me right up to the end.

STRUGGLING TO STAY CONNECTED

I have learned that it is one thing to forget things or forget people, but forgetting how to speak is quite another. Speech is one of humanity's most distinguishing characteristics. It's how we connect and interrelate with those around us, how we make friends and interact with the world.

As children, we learn speech slowly over many years and, as we acquire more words, our ability to interact in a meaningful way with friends and family also increases. In Mike's case, the opposite occurred. As time went on, he was slowly losing his words, and I began to realize that, if we were not careful, he would also lose his ability to connect with those he loved.

In the beginning, when Mike first started having difficulty with words, we saw a speech therapist at the local hospital. She was kind and helpful in her own way, but her suggestions were too complicated for Mike, so we did the best we could on our own.

Each passing month saw new declines in Mike's speech (see my journal entries later in this chapter). At first it was a missing word here and there, then sentences without a subject, which left me guessing the topic. Fortunately, during the early years of the illness, because we had been married forever and had a lifetime of shared experiences, I could usually fill in the blanks and figure out what he was saying. Later, when language was gone, his facial expressions, gestures, touches and eyes were how we communicated.

LEARNING NEW WAYS TO COMMUNICATE

Two years before Mike passed away, our dear longtime friend Shirley, a speech therapist, came from California for a visit. We had such a good time, visiting the lavender farm, picking blackberries, and oh, yes, making and eating blackberry pie.

The night before she departed I asked Mike, "Can we talk to Shirley about your speech?" He said yes, and in the morning the three of us sat at the dining room table and had a visit.

Shirley really grasped the difficulty of the problem and was so good at listening, understanding, and then suggesting different ways for Mike to say something, including: if you cannot get the word out, then come at it from a different direction; use substitute words you know for words you no longer know; use photo albums and picture books; point to pictures of food so you can show Rosalys what you want to eat. Most of all, she urged Mike to keep talking, just keep communicating in any way you can—and never give up.

So that is what Mike and I decided to do. We went with what our friend Shirley said and just kept Mike talking, pointing or communicating any way he could.

I could usually understand what Mike wanted to tell me, but it might take multiple techniques. I might point at things so he could say yes or no. Or I might ask my son or daughter when they were present to try and figure out what Dad wanted. Or I might suggest we take a break and try figuring it out later.

Quite frankly, as time progressed, there were some conversations that I hoped would just go away. And there were more than a few times when I would simply praise Mike's effort to communicate and act like I got what he was trying to say, even though I did not have a clue, for that was the best I could do.

In the beginning, Mike would get frustrated when I couldn't understand him, but over time he just decided not to let this get to him. He simply refused to get upset by difficult conversations. After multiple attempts at trying to get me to understand something, he would just shake his head or raise his hand, indicating, "Enough!"—he was done with it. He had made the decision early on not to let the language problem get to him, and that is exactly what he did—amazing!

Because of Mike, I learned that communication doesn't always require a mutual exchange. I remember one time driving along with Mike and he was talking about something. I kept nodding and grabbing a word here and there, but honestly I had no idea what he was trying to say. I noticed that there was no expression on his face that indicated it was something important that he really wanted me to get. So, instead of trying to get him to repeat or explain (as I had done in the past), this time I just thought: this is working pretty well; so I just enjoyed the pleasure of a visit with Mike as I drove and he talked.

I never did figure out what he was saying that day, so I couldn't respond, but we were still communicating in our own way. My nodding appreciatively signified that Mike still had things to tell me, and that I cared for him and wanted to listen. That was communication too.

As my journal entries show below, Mike's ability to communicate continued to decline, year by year—but there is a ray of sunlight in our experience: Through it all, we never gave up, and we both found ways to communicate our love for each other, even at the very end of the journey.

⤙ FROM MY JOURNAL ⤚

YEAR ONE

A week or so ago we had words over what Mike was doing the next day. He had multiple tasks for the church and house. I was checking to be sure he had the time figured out. He was angry because I was interfering. Within a short time he got back to me to explain he was angry because he couldn't explain all the things he was going to do. He knew what he had to do but could not express it to me.

⁓

*He also explained how he couldn't fill in the parts of a TV show
I had missed. He said, "You have no idea how hard it is to talk
with someone and not be able to say the words you want." We need
social time but don't want the setting to be difficult for Mike.*

~

*I find I make so many mistakes with words—I am not sure if I just
notice them or if I am getting affected by association. Sister Patty
will be here on Saturday; I am really ready to talk with her. She
will be a good person to assess how we are progressing.*

~

*Mike forgot a word last night, so we talked a bit. He has chosen
not to go to the Customs Christmas party this year. He also said
he would take care of things at the house while I went alone to a
neighbor's open house. I said I thought it was because he forgets
words—he agreed.*

~

*I feel like I talk a lot when in a group and jump in to correct or
finish Mike's story. I need to watch that.*

~

*We went to a neighborhood meeting in Montana. Mike said after-
wards it's sad not to be able to join in the conversation. The words
just don't come to him. He knows what he wants to say. He said he
can only join in in a lighthearted manner*

~

*Need to remember not to get angry at little things— like having to
repeat something or restate something different (for Mike).*

YEAR TWO

*Mike is having increased trouble remembering words. Once again,
it is a reminder to be realistic. I need to ask if he has said what he
wants to say to people.*

~

When I ask for clarification about something, it is upsetting to Mike. Better not to ask right then. Later he seems to come back to it and not get upset over my asking for information.

~

Mike has been talking about Christmas. He wants to get Pat a stylish hat and Kathleen a tool belt. Mike gives me daily "I love yous" and frequently says "Goodnight Sweetheart" (my favorite). I continue to be so lucky having Mike in my life. We have the time to say and do what is important to us.

YEAR THREE

Lots of words missing and incorrect, uses wrong tense. Said NPT for NPR. Makes similar mistakes, often.

~

It's great to have Patrick around. While Pat and I were cooking, Mike said that he (Mike) was a 'superferlus' man… (so)… Pat put him right to work peeling carrots.

~

Mike's sentence structure is more difficult to follow, loses more words and doesn't understand why I don't know what he is saying. In the afternoon, on our way home from Montana, there was no back-and-forth conversation. I would put out a "bid" and get no response or I needed to repeat 3 or 4 times. Cannot seem to see things when I point. I point right and he looks left.

~

Mike frequently wants me to tell someone something that he cannot: "Tell Ellie about the sodas." Problem is I don't always know what he is talking about. In this case 'soda' was about tooth decay and fluoride.

~

Mike is having more trouble remembering words. Once again it is a reminder to be "realistic." (This isn't going away.) I want to ask him if he has said the things he wants to say to people. I'm not sure that is a good idea.

~

I am so glad we did Mike's life story video last May, I don't think Mike now could say the things he said then.

YEAR FOUR

It is more difficult for him to tell me his thoughts, things in the newspaper or just ideas—important for me to always come if he has something to tell me.

~

Mike said: "We have to figure out how I can communicate with you." He talked about speech lessons.

~

A few weeks ago, I repeated something three times and then was a little irritable about it. Mike put his arms around me and said "I don't mean to be a burden to you." He gave me such a nice hug— what more could I want.

YEAR FIVE
(See chapter 29: What Our Life was Like in Year 5)

~

YEAR SIX

Mike's ability to tell me what he needs is still possible but difficult. Usually even a few words and I can get it. "Kathleen... dollars... give her." He was talking about the silver dollars we found a month ago. It is hard for me to watch Mike try to converse with others and not be able to... but he doesn't get angry.

~

On our way to Stan's, Mike said, "I just wish I could talk."

YEAR 7

The last few days I have felt so sad for Michael. His ability to speak is so limited. I find myself crying as I write, which is one of the first times for me to have tears.

~

Newspaper helps. Mike can show me things of interest. Telling something to friends seems impossible now. It is so hard to watch him struggle.

~

Mike is slipping and yet he is still Mike. We communicate, but I don't usually know what he is telling me. I get his love pats, but his thoughts are not clear. Talked about his brother while in the kitchen with my neighbor and me. "My brother... he was here." Mike does not have a brother. I think it must have been about Bob (my brother-in-law.)

YEAR 8
(18 MONTHS BEFORE MIKE DIED)

Mike currently very emotionally connected. When I was going to call my sister Patty, he said: "Tell her I love her." When I was on my hands and knees cleaning up spilled coffee, he said: "You look like the ba ba baby, but bigger." We had a good laugh together.

(17 MONTHS BEFORE HE DIED)

Last night, Mike was tucked into bed and as I started to leave he said, "Honey." I returned and knelt beside the bed. "I love you." The words were said so clear, just like he used to always say them. Those words are so powerful and what makes this all so easy.

~

During the day, I told Mike about an unpleasant email I received about work. He asked about it again before bed: "Your work?" I got it and said it worked out.

(13 MONTHS BEFORE HE DIED)

Mike took a bedroom spill when he got up from his nap. Kathleen and I were unable to get him up so called the paramedics. They did it quick and easy. Before they left, Mike patted the paramedic's hand and said "Thank you."

~

Two nights ago, Mike wet the bed. We got up at 5:00 and I changed the bed. He sat in the chair and when we got back in bed he said "Thank you." So few words and yet he says the important ones. I still get "I lov lov you."

~

Yesterday was Mike's 75th birthday. A perfect day with a small group of friends and family, even our group of 23 was a lot for Mike. He did fine. At one point he was able to convey to me that he couldn't talk to them. I told him it was okay, I would talk for us.

~

Mike did communicate (at his birthday). Played harmonica, smiled, and talked like Donald Duck. He also danced—while sitting—to a musical birthday card. It is amazing how well he still communicates and yet cannot really talk.

(TEN MONTHS BEFORE HE DIED)

Patrick stayed with Mike for two nights, while I went to Victoria with my sisters. When I returned Patrick and I had a valuable conversation about so many things, including death and dying. He also told me that his dad wanted to see his friends and that perhaps a party would be nice. Amazing that Patrick and Mike were able to have a conversation of that depth. We had a party!

(SIX MONTHS BEFORE HE DIED)

This morning when I awoke, I said "Hi." Mike could not respond with "Hi" back. It made me cry. When I think about what this must be like for Mike, I'm very sad.

~

Mike is speaking less:
"Thank you"
"Hi"
"I lovve yim"
"Water"
Makes funny faces and expresses emotions with face. Lets me
know when he has had enough to eat. Mumbles, doesn't have full
sentences with missing nouns like he used to.

~

A difficult Saturday, I changed Mike three times, then complained.
"This is the third change—I'm tired." Mike began to cry. I told him
how sorry I was and would not complain to him again, and that he
is doing the hard work and never complains. He doesn't deserve me
complaining and I will not do it again. "I am so sorry."
It is so unfair to complain to him. He can't fight back,
his only defense was to cry—so sad.

(ONE MONTH BEFORE MIKE DIED)

Once again there is a shift. We have moved from a quiet time to
a more restless time. Lots of calling, yelling, and crying when he
wakes and when tired. I need to remember all of the above are how
he calls me or tells me he needs something, and in fact be glad he is
still communicating.

WHEN MIKE TALKED TO STRANGERS

Before we leave this chapter, here are two tender moments that occurred in Year 5 of Mike's illness when he attempted to talk to strangers.

One was with a hotshot smoke jumper on the train from Montana to Seattle. I began the conversation with this older man and soon Mike joined in with a nod or a smile and, eventually, some simple questions.

The smoke jumper had wonderful stories and was eager to share, and Mike was a good listener. It seemed to be going so well that I excused myself for a quick bathroom break. When I returned, I could see things had fallen apart. The man was no longer talking, and Mike looked sad. It seemed that while I had stepped away, the conversation had turned from the detailed stories we had enjoyed about fighting fires, to questions from the man about what Mike did for a living. Clearly, that conversation was impossible for Mike to engage in without my help.

It was disappointing to see Mike's sadness when I returned. On the bright side, however, Mike had enjoyed most of that conversation with a stranger. He had enjoyed hearing another person's life story. He was delighted that the stranger hadn't looked at him as "different"—that he had simply valued Mike as an equal. I loved watching Mike join in on the conversation and respond in all the right ways to this man. Carrying on a simple conversation is something we all take for granted.

Another conversation with a stranger occurred with a volunteer at the Spruce Goose Museum in McMinnville, Oregon. After completing the museum tour, Mike wanted to know who ran the museum and went back in to find out. I tagged along knowing he would not be able to ask the question.

Much to my surprise, Mike didn't need my help with this particular conversation after all. I wondered why and realized it was probably because the volunteer was older, talked slowly, and processed Mike's questions slowly, too, which all worked for Mike. This bright conversant senior was perfect for Mike, answering questions slowly and thoughtfully and picking up on Mike's facial expressions for more detail. The man had no idea I was watching and learning from him, or that Mike had Alzheimer's.

And then there were the social events with our circle of friends and acquaintances. Initially, Mike avoided these because he didn't want everyone to see his struggles with Alzheimer's. As time went by, however, he was willing to attend because everyone knew of his limitations and had made adjustments to make him feel comfortable.

They knew, for example, that they should carry most of the conversation for Mike and could look to me to fill in the blanks.

As time went on, I found myself carrying more and more of the conversation for Mike and me. Still, Mike loved these moments. He liked to be part of the discussion, even when he could no longer converse.

Some helpful thoughts on managing those open conversations with others: When you are with someone who has Alzheimer's, help your loved one join in on the conversation as much as possible. Bring them right into the conversation, and help tell their story with them and for them. And continue to refer to them by name throughout the conversation, so they can nod or make a face about the funny event that you share.

Don't leave your loved one alone in a social situation, for he/she will surely end up isolated from the people who want to include him or her, but who cannot do it without your help.

INSIGHTS

- Long after Mike had lost most of his vocabulary, he continued to amaze me with his awareness of the world around him. His words were failing him, but he was still Mike, still there with us in our family, and still connected to the important parts of our lives.

WHAT MIKE DID AND HOW HE DID IT:

- Put himself out there, and continued to interact in the world the best he could.
- Looked at me when he needed help in a conversation.
- Used the newspaper to point out things of interest to share a thought.
- Verbally said, "I love you" to those who were important to him as long as possible.
- Later said, "I love you" with his eyes.
- Used humor and laughter, saw the lighter side.

- Late in the disease, he created laughter by using a Donald Duck voice or moving his eyebrows up and down like Groucho Marx.
- Played the harmonica or whistled.
- Shook his head to tell me I had it wrong, or smiled when I had it right.
- Kept his calm and took a break whenever necessary.

WHAT I DID:

- Tried to keep in mind how difficult this must be for Mike.
- Listened when he wanted to talk about the difficulty and told him I knew it was really hard.
- Told him often what a good job he was doing communicating.
- Later, I became his voice and told others what he liked and did not like. And even verbalized his feelings when I thought I knew them.
- Created a photo album with pictures of friends and family. It helped for me to point to people if he was attempting to tell me something about someone, and also served to prompt him before someone came.
- Used a photo album to show him food, which was not as helpful as we hoped. (Perhaps we tried this too late.)
- Learned to remain patient, pausing often to give him time to process words or information.
- Learned not to jump into his conversation when it was not necessary.
- Focused on what Mike said, and valued what he said.
- Stayed calm, and encouraged a break when we needed it.
- Refrained from using the word "DON'T." I helped Mike by communicating what to do rather than what not to do.
- Used simple sentences, such as, "Lift your foot."
- Included him in conversations I had with others.
- Talked with him about his day, my day, and our day.
- Pointed a lot, giving him visual cues for food, clothes, directions, etc.
- Used pointing to show him the sky, flowers, clouds and, of course, our favorite, the moon. And he returned the favor in kind. A big full moon shining in our bedroom was a treasured cue for him to point at something we both loved.

LAST BUT NOT LEAST:

- Remember your loved one may not have the words to tell you something, but he or she knows more than you might think.

- Keep laughter alive.

- Talk to strangers.

- Never give up—just keep communicating any way you can.

CHAPTER 25

TABLE FOR TWO

*As time went on, the pleasant
tradition of eating together became
more and more of a challenge for us.
What to do?*

FOOD IS SUSTENANCE FOR THE BODY, and its preparation and enjoyment are sustenance for your relationship. With or without Alzheimer's, sharing meals together is important. It's how we celebrate holidays and events, how we create memories with each other, and how we identify with our family roots and who we are.

As Mike's journey with Alzheimer's continued, the pleasant tradition of eating together became more and more of a chore. As it turned out, by making a few changes in how, when and where we ate, Mike and I were able to continue to dine together, to enjoy sharing meals with friends and family, and to preserve Mike's dignity while dining.

WHAT SOUNDS GOOD FOR DINNER?

It's an age-old ritual: When mealtime rolls around, we ask our loved one, "What sounds good for dinner?" When we go to the store to buy groceries, we ask, "Is there something special I can pick up for you?" When we go out to a restaurant, we ask, "What are you thinking about ordering?"

But, as time wore on, Mike's words began to fail him and he had real difficulty answering these routine questions. This was stressful for me and embarrassing for Mike. I knew we had to figure this one out, and we did. Here are some of the ways we did it:

- Whenever possible Mike and I went to the grocery store together so Mike could actually show me the items he wanted.
- We also tried using a photo album with pictures of food. The idea was that Mike would simply point to the items he wanted (no language necessary), and I would prepare those items or pick them up at the store for him. In practice this didn't always work for Mike because he didn't think the pictures looked like the food we ate. But it's worth a try with your loved one.
- Before going out to a restaurant, Mike and I would sit down at home and decide in advance what we planned to order. Since restaurants have similar basic categories (pasta, chicken, fish, hamburger, salad, vegetables, etc.) you don't really need a menu to choose your basic preference. When we arrived at the restaurant I would simply remind Mike of what he had decided at home and place the order for him from the closest things on the menu.

While all of the above helped for a time, there was one thing that helped right up to the very end: I knew which foods Mike loved! By knowing Mike's favorite foods and making a few changes, we avoided those long silences where the server is waiting for answers to their questions—which again helped preserve Mike's dignity.

MAKING FRIENDS WITH FINGER FOODS

When Mike could no longer use utensils, I thought about young children and how we make it possible for them to feed themselves. The same techniques worked well for Mike too.

Just like when our kids were young, Mike and I avoided fancy restaurants at night. Early lunch or dinner, especially at less formal restaurants, worked fine.

Finger foods became our friends, including peanut butter and jelly, grilled cheese sandwiches, crackers and cheese, soft cooked carrot sticks, asparagus, broccoli, sliced oranges, pears, chicken— all were foods that Mike enjoyed and were easy for him to pick up with his fingers.

Two pottery pieces were incredibly helpful. First, a mug with no handle made it possible for him to drink coffee unassisted for a long time. (The handle on a cup was difficult for him to manage.) Second, a bowl with a handle allowed Mike to hang on to it while he used a large spoon (so the bowl no longer moved on the table).

Occasionally Mike ate with a napkin tucked in his shirt collar, but we never had to resort to a bib because his food was simple.

ENJOYING MEALS WITH OTHERS

Sharing meals with friends and family was important to us so we continued to invite friends to our home for dinner and continued to say "yes" to celebrations and events when invited.

People seemed to understand Mike's challenge and served meals that worked pretty well for us. There were always some finger foods that Mike could hold and manage by himself. And, if he needed help with food on a fork, I could always help out with that.

At these "friends and family" get-togethers I could easily talk and visit with people at the table as I helped Mike manage his food, and he enjoyed the interaction with friends, smiling and laughing with everyone else when funny stories were told.

I remember fondly attending our St. Barnabas Supper Club group eight years after Mike was diagnosed. This was a Sunday afternoon group of six women and Mike. We had such a good time going to each of the different women's homes that year. The host would often call ahead to make sure the menu would work for Mike and would ask how Mike was doing. Everyone was so kind even when something spilled or a cup was broken.

CONTINUING OUR DINNERS FOR TWO

For years Mike and I had shared our meals together as often as possible, and we didn't want Alzheimer's to interfere with that. Throughout the early and middle years of Mike's illness I would set up dinner at the large dining room table. There we would sit down, as always, and enjoy a leisurely dinner for two and conversation. I felt it was important and comforting for us to continue this old and pleasant ritual as long as possible.

Even in Mike's final year of life we were able to dine together at home. That last year I did move our dinner to a smaller table in the living room and usually turned on the evening TV news. The little table was much easier to set up, and the news helped me carry on a conversation with Mike now that he spoke so little.

Eventually some meals were shared in bed—breakfast in the morning or a favorite snack at night, for example. The time and place for our meal might change but, despite Alzheimer's, we continued to dine together as a couple.

SAVOR THE MOMENT

Year after year Mike and I looked forward to holiday meals and celebrations. For all we knew they might be coming to an end at any time, but Mike's motto was "enjoy the moment" and we did just that.

His final year of life was no exception. Despite his continuing decline, there was Christmas and Easter and then Mike's birthday to celebrate—all with his favorite foods.

On May 23rd Mike turned 76, just two weeks before he died, and even then we had a party—a simple celebration—with our good friends Stan and Audrey. They filled our bedroom with smiles and laughter as the sun poured in the window.

Later we had an unexpected surprise when our neighbors Gary and Linda and their daughter Signe arrived with helium birthday balloons and big smiles—it was perfect! They, too, joined us for a little of Mike's favorite dessert—pineapple upside down cake. I took photos on that beautiful spring day, and Mike's expression was one of contentment.

Today, the grandchildren and I still enjoy making grandpa Mike's favorite cake to commemorate his birthday every May 23rd. They love measuring the flour, pineapple and cherry pieces, and delight in hearing stories and memories about Grandpa Mike.

So Mike stayed in our life with shared meals and celebrations right up to the very last weeks of his illness, and now he is still part of our life because of the memories we created and the food he loved.

CHAPTER 26

MAKING THE MOST
OF MEDICATIONS

*How I helped Mike manage the
effectiveness of his prescriptions.*

WHEN MIKE WAS FIRST DIAGNOSED, his doctor explained to us that no medications had yet been developed to stop or cure Alzheimer's disease. That was true then, and it's still true as I write this.

I'm confident that a cure will be discovered, either quite soon or in the foreseeable future. Until then, however, we must turn to medications that are proven to help some patients delay the worst effects of the disease.

As Mike's doctor explained to us, these medications tend to be expensive, and they can vary in effectiveness from one person to another. Each individual must assess with his/her own doctor the advantages and disadvantages of taking any particular drug. In our case, neither Mike nor I hesitated. If there was a medication that gave reasonable hope of improving his abilities for a time, we wanted our doctor to prescribe it for him.

Over the course of Mike's illness he relied on three different Alzheimer's medications. Each new medication was started with a low dose and gradually increased to minimize any side effects. Mike adjusted to each new medication without much difficulty.

Aricept was the first medication he tried, and the improvement in his condition was both quick and dramatic. With Aricept it was almost as if the old Mike was back. In no time he was more engaged and communicating better. This little pill was our friend for years, just as it is for many Alzheimer's couples today.

Mike used all the significant medications that were available for Alzheimer's at the time. Each one improved his abilities for a while and then gradually became less effective. Mike's doctor continued to monitor his cognitive abilities with neurological tests, always asking how he was functioning to determine if his current medication and dose were effective and then made the necessary changes as needed.

HELPFUL TIPS FOR THE CAREGIVER

Over the years I learned simple ways to help Mike leverage the effectiveness of the various medications he was taking. By working closely with your doctor, you, too, can evaluate whether these or similar tips can help you and your loved one get the best results from your medications:

1. **Give pills on time and with food.** By far the most important discipline was to *always* give the medication on time and to *always* ensure there was food in Mike's stomach before taking a pill. That may sound obvious, but it's easy for a busy spouse/caregiver to run late with the medication or forget to give it with food.

2. **Use a numbered pillbox.** I soon learned the importance of a weekly pillbox that I could fill each Monday and then watch the number go down each day. There were days I would discover I missed a pill and felt terrible, but with a busy life at home it happens. It's up to the spouse/caregiver to minimize those oversights and the numbered pillbox helped.

3. **Keep snacks on hand.** Whenever you leave the house together and might have to take a pill on the road, take a snack with you. Mike's favorite by far was half a peanut butter and jelly sandwich. The sandwich was easy for him to hold, gave him enough food so he could have a pill, and there was no refrigeration needed. When traveling in the car I always took bread, peanut butter and jelly. Simple.

4. **Learn to refine your timing.** While it is important to always give medication on time, you can make small adjustments in your schedule to improve the pill's effectiveness even more. For example, I learned that there was a significant *decrease* in Mike's abilities as he neared the time for another pill—just as there was a significant *increase* in his abilities 30 minutes to an hour after taking a pill. And so I adjusted breakfast and dinner to get the best possible advantage out of the medication.

By the end of Mike's ninth year I made a number of important changes. Breakfast pills stayed at the same time, but I learned to give him breakfast in bed, pills, a nap, and then get him up. That gave an hour or so for the medication to work which made getting him out of bed oh-so-much easier.

A year or so earlier, I had made a similar adjustment for dinner. I started giving him a light 4:00 P.M. snack, followed by his pills. That made the dinner hour so much easier and more interactive. Waiting for pills until 5:00 P.M. or 6:00 P.M. was just too long.

A WORD ABOUT LATE-STAGE MEDICATIONS

Towards the end of Mike's illness, Lorazepam was prescribed. It can be given in pill form under the tongue and can be used to relax a person, promote sleep, or help with pain.

I was advised that Mike would build up a tolerance to Lorazepam and would need the medication every two hours to help him sleep. That did not seem helpful to me. If I had to wake up to give him medication every two hours, then how would either one of us get any decent sleep? So I gave it to him sparingly and it worked out fine.

When hospice joined our circle, we were told it was no longer necessary for Mike to use his Alzheimer's medication. We considered that advice, but it seemed to me that the medication was still helping him—so we continued using it anyway.

During the final weeks of his illness, when he was eating very little, Mike had some distress that we could not pin down. He seemed to have pain, but what was it from? I finally concluded it might be due to his taking medication while only having a small amount of food in his stomach. At that point we finally halted medication.

Some will argue that medication is not helpful when a person is in the late stage of Alzheimer's. That was not so for Mike. As I have mentioned throughout this book, he continued to function quite well throughout the ninth year. I am confident that that would not have been possible without the aid of medication.

NOTE: Please check with your own doctor before you make any decisions regarding medications.

⟶ FROM MY JOURNAL ⟵
JANUARY (YEAR 8)

This was a difficult day—Mike just did not have it together. He didn't have a clue what I was talking about. I would say lift your foot and he would lift his arm. It turned out I missed his morning pills—he got them at noon. Kathleen said what a difference when she picked him up from Stan's at 4:00 P.M.—he was really good—talking and everything.

──────────────── **INSIGHTS** ────────────────

- Although current medications cannot cure Alzheimer's or stop it from progressing, we know that they may help lessen symptoms, such as memory loss and confusion, for a limited time.

- In Mike's case, I am confident that his medication made a significant difference in my ability to care for him at home.

- I learned that there is a variable in how effective medication is for each individual, and I gained a new appreciation of our Doctor's regular assessments of Mike's neurological abilities. Meanwhile, I could help to assess Mike's abilities by simply noting how he functioned when he was with me. Working together with Mike's doctor, we made the best medication choices for Mike.

- When a person is taken off Alzheimer's medication, there is typically a significant immediate dip in their abilities. In other words, the medication does not have a long-term effect.

- When Mike could no longer swallow pills, I was told that I could open the capsule and give him the medication with some water, which worked. I wish I had asked about this sooner. Again, ask your doctor.

- During the last weeks of Mike's life I kept a notebook beside his bed. This made it easy for the caregivers and me to share notes on how much he ate and when medication was given.

- Most Alzheimer's patients typically go off medication once they are in hospice; but my experience was that keeping Mike on medication as long as possible (even in hospice) worked to his advantage.

CHAPTER 27

MAINTAINING YOUR PARTNER'S DIGNITY

Alzheimer's does its best to rob
people of their dignity—but it
doesn't have to be that way.

As ALZHEIMER'S PROGRESSES your loved one will naturally find it more and more difficult to manage everyday routines such as getting dressed or using the bathroom. But Mike and I were both determined that he would stay in charge of his own life as much as possible and maintain his dignity as long as possible.

Looking back, I think we did a pretty good job of it. Here are some of the ways we managed:

STRIPED SHIRTS AND PLAID PANTS?

The Mike I knew and loved was always well-groomed. In his job with U.S. Customs he was a suit-and-tie guy for years and always looked sharp as he walked out the door in the morning.

When he retired, Mike made the switch to casual pants and button-down shirts, still neat and clean but a more casual look. Later, when Alzheimer's came along, I naturally wanted to jump right in and help him stay well-groomed. But I also knew he wanted to dress himself as long as possible, without me or anyone else micromanaging.

Hmm, how do you stand quietly by if your loved one picks a striped shirt to wear with his plaid pants; or selects a warm sweater on a hot day; or forgets a jacket when it's raining? Or is struggling to get dressed? At what point do you insert yourself in the process?

My daughter helped me with this when she suggested, "Ask Dad if he needs help." What a novel idea—ask instead of just jumping in. So, from that point on, I would ask Mike if he needed help and, if he did, he would say so. If he didn't, then I would just leave the room and trust him to make his best decisions.

JUST ENOUGH, BUT NOT TOO MUCH

As Alzheimer's progressed and it really did become necessary to help Mike get dressed, I helped him "just enough but not too much." It's the same principle I used when our children were young. I helped them by pulling up their slacks part way or starting their shirt over their head, but then allowing them to finish the task themselves. And when they did, I always praised them by affirming, "Great job, you did it!"

And that is what I did with Mike too. Even if he could only help a little by lifting his foot for his shoe or pushing his arm through a sleeve, I let him complete the task himself and then praised him for the effort. This gave him the same sense of accomplishment that all of us need to keep going and feel relevant in life.

On a purely practical note, I eventually made a few adjustments in Mike's wardrobe, which made it easier for him to remain independent as long as possible. Instead of jeans and belts, for example, we chose sweats with drawstrings or pants with elastic waistbands. Mike's favorite jacket had a zipper and loose sleeves. His shirts had to have wide openings at the top and no buttons. And the best footwear was slip-on shoes and loose socks.

The bottom line was that Mike's new clothing made it easier for him to continue dressing himself, and he still felt well-groomed and well-dressed. These simple basics helped to preserve his dignity and self-esteem. There were no complaints from Mike because, by then, we were both ready for any reasonable compromise that kept our lives as normal and easy as possible.

FRIENDS AND FAMILY HELPED

Helping dress someone is a whole different level of intimacy for both parties—something that is not for everyone. If I were present, Mike always preferred that I help him get dressed. But eventually it was necessary to ask certain family members and friends to help.

It all worked out, though. Somehow, our loving family members and friends each found a way of making it seem like it was no big deal. And, of course, the professional caregivers were just that—professional—and managed to keep Mike's dignity in all that they did.

There were, however, certain situations that required a little extra creativity. What would you do, for example, if you were out in public and needed to help your loved one with personal clothing or bathroom needs? At first, I spent many concerned moments outside men's restrooms wondering if Mike was doing okay inside. I did everything from asking strangers to check on him to marching right in myself when it seemed all the men were out.

Eventually, as Mike's needs increased and I got wiser, I simply used the women's restroom with him and it was not a problem. We would go in when I saw it was not busy and call out that I was coming in with my husband who needed a little help. We used an accessible stall and I simply called out to anyone who entered that I was in the end stall helping my husband. This technique was never a problem and the women were quite gracious. By working together in these ways, Mike's dignity was preserved and we never had a clothing or bathroom problem in public.

~ FROM MY JOURNAL ~
JANUARY (YEAR 5)

Dressing is becoming difficult for Mike. Puts slacks on backwards and has to start over. He doesn't like me to help him with his jacket. Puts underwear on backwards and sometimes two legs in one side. He hangs in there and gets it done—slowly. I love him.

APRIL (YEAR 6)

He needs help with slacks and shirt after restroom, but smiles and puts up with help I give him. There are bigger dips in ups and downs now. Sometimes dresses self well and other times he has a lot of difficulty.

JUNE (YEAR 6)

Mike is so appreciative. He works and works at something and then I'll check in and help him or he will come looking for me. The other day I was at my desk and I heard "Rosie." Here came Mike needing his shirt buttoned. "I just need a few." Didn't want me to have to do them all. We continue to hug and kiss a lot—how lucky I am.

JANUARY (YEAR 7)

Mike can still let me know what he wants—his glasses, different shoes, his hat, his gloves—it is usually difficult but we figure it out.

INSIGHTS

- With all the demands that Alzheimer's puts on people, it might be tempting to let everyday grooming slip—but Mike and I were careful not to let that happen.

- When he started needing a little more help, I laid his clothes out and put them in the order he would want them, and then allowed him to dress himself, with a little help from me here and there.

- Helping a grown man with jeans is difficult. Year 7 is when we started using slacks with elastic—a most excellent change!

- I learned to be patient and give him lots of time. For Mike to continue feeling successful he needed more time to complete routine tasks that were now complicated for him.

- The very act of being up, dressed and out of bed each day has a lot to do with how we feel about ourselves and how others view us. Despite Alzheimer's, Mike was up, looked tidy, and ready for the day even the last few weeks of his life—and that made all the difference in the quality of his days.

- Good advice for all couples: "Catch your partner doing something right and praise them for it." I always tried to remember this with Mike, especially when he worked so hard at everyday tasks such as dressing himself.

- A note about using Depends®: Yes disposable underwear did enter our life, but not until the ninth year. Some think that when Depends® are needed they can no longer care for their loved one at home. That is something each individual will have to decide, but it turned out that Depends® were not a big problem for Mike and me. As always, I simply sat down and explained to him that in order for us to continue dealing with Alzheimer's at home it would be necessary to use Depends®, and he was agreeable.

CHAPTER 28

THE MAGIC OF PROPER SLEEP

*By carefully managing Mike's sleep
patterns we made it possible for him
to function at a higher level.*

IF MIKE DID NOT GET ENOUGH SLEEP AT NIGHT, or if we skipped his scheduled naps during the day, he became agitated and confused. Everyone knows that agitation and confusion are common symptoms of Alzheimer's disease, but I'm convinced that the simple lack of sleep may be a bigger contributor to those symptoms than people realize.

To put it more positively, consider this: by carefully managing Mike's evening sleep and daily naps, I believe we minimized the usual irritability associated with this disease, and improved his ability to function at a higher level for an extended time.

While sleep requirements vary from person to person, I can safely guarantee that if you and your loved one figure out how to get the sleep you both need, it will make a dramatic difference in your entire Alzheimer's journey.

To that end, here are some simple ways that Mike and I learned to get the required sleep for our daily challenges with Alzheimer's:

WATCH FOR YOUR LOVED ONE'S
CHANGING SLEEP NEEDS

In Chapter 1, I mentioned that just before Mike was diagnosed with Alzheimer's he was told that he had sleep apnea. His doctor prescribed a CPAP machine which decreased his snoring, and Mike slept soundly for quite a while after that.

During the first couple years of Alzheimer's, he continued to sleep through the night, but, as time went on, I noticed certain changes. He began nodding off more and more during the day. He often fell asleep in the car when we were out for a drive, and he would typically nod off while he watched the evening news and I prepared dinner. At first I thought this might be depression, but his doctor said that she did not think that was the case.

I began to get impatient when Mike wanted to sleep during the best parts of the day, and he would sometimes get cranky with me in return. I wondered: "What's really going on in Mike's body and mind—and how can we make it better for him and for us?"

Then one day it dawned on me. I was teaching one of my classes for new parents and we were discussing how important it is for parents to monitor their baby's changing sleep requirements. Typically, little newborns need to sleep a great deal. Later, they can get by on a routine of two naps a day. Later still, they need just one scheduled nap per day, but they will become very agitated and fussy if they don't get that nap.

"Aha," I thought, "this is what's happening with Mike too. His sleep needs are changing, much like an infant's, except in reverse. As an infant grows and matures, he or she needs fewer naps and less sleep. But with Alzheimer's patients, the process works in the opposite direction. With Alzheimer's you slowly lose basic abilities such as language, balance and memory. Some refer to this decline as "going back in time." It turns out that in our case it also applied to sleep. As Alzheimer's progressed, Mike gradually moved back toward an earlier developmental stage and, like a newborn, required more sleep. No one told us that might happen!

START REGULATING DAILY NAPS

Now that I understood the principle, it was easier to anticipate and plan for Mike's increasing sleep requirements. It took a little convincing, but Mike soon got on board with the idea of formal naps.

At first we scheduled a one-hour nap each afternoon, right after lunch. This nap was good for me, too. While he was sleeping I could move freely about the house without being "on" for Mike—a welcome break!

As Alzheimer's progressed, I could see that a single nap was no longer enough, so we added a second nap, this one in the early morning. It worked like this: Mike would wake at 9:00 A.M. and have breakfast; a couple of hours later he would take his first nap of the day. I would wake him for lunch and, after lunch, we would go for a drive or an outing and then come back for his afternoon nap.

Just as a mother learns to maintain a regular nap routine for her child, I learned the importance of keeping Mike's daily nap routine consistent. They were always at the same time of day, always in our bedroom, always in the same position, shoes off, curtains closed and the door cracked. Later I found wonderful lullaby music— the *Songs of Innocence* by Julie Anne Meixsell—that was perfect. I would turn on the soothing lullabies and Mike would drift right off.

REGULATE EVENING BEDTIME TOO

It was a nice surprise that we did not need to rely on sleep medication to help Mike sleep at night. When his routine bedtime rolled around he was more than ready to sleep and usually dozed all through the night. This was a blessing for both of us.

There were exceptions, of course. During the last few months of Mike's life he awoke frequently, just as a newborn might. For this I responded with a new and soothing ritual that we both liked. He would awaken, I would change him if needed, sit him up, and tell him I would be right back with a milkshake. I came up with the milkshake idea because Mike's weight was going down and it was difficult to give him enough calories during the day.

Those are fond memories. We would sit contentedly—Mike in bed and me in a comfy chair beside him—and just talk a little about life while giving him sips of milkshake. Then Mike would settle back into his favorite sleeping position. A lullaby would be turned on and the lights turned off. Hopefully, we both went back to sleep. Mike usually did, but I often didn't.

CAREGIVERS NEED SLEEP TOO!

It's often said that a patient will only do as well as his or her caregiver does. I think there's some truth in that.

If the caregiver does not get enough sleep then everything else begins to unravel, including your physical health, your attitude, and your ability to care for your loved one in a patient and compassionate way. So you simply must make your own sleep a priority.

I managed pretty well as long as I got a nap during the day. I learned to nap when Mike napped and to let the housework and other tasks go. I took twenty-minute naps on the ferry on my way to work, as well as catnaps when someone else was caring for Mike.

Whenever I taught my weekend workshops I had one or two restful and wonderful nights away from home. Knowing Mike was in good hands, I could catch up on my sleep with no worries. If you are the caregiver, I highly recommend a periodic night or two away for you too.

It is easy to say that caregivers need their sleep, but it is not always easy to do. Here is a journal note that captures the struggle I had in heeding my own advice.

⟶ FROM MY JOURNAL ⟵
YEAR EIGHT

I am surprised how little I can get done other than care for Mike. We returned from Montana a month ago and I have not had time to even sweep the driveway. Because my only free time is his nap time, sweeping the driveway is low on the list. Alas it is a busy time, but basically we continue to have fun and laugh a lot. Thank you Michael!

- Mike and I were sometimes short with each other, but I now think it was usually due to fatigue. Get sleep any way you can—don't ever put it at the bottom of your list.

- If you take a nap during the day, you will discover you are a better care-giver late in the afternoon and night.

- Studies indicate that sleep disturbance occurs in about half to three quarters of those with Alzheimer's. Once I started to think of Mike's increasing need for sleep as a normal process, everything made more sense. And it certainly led to improving our dispositions.

- Many who have Alzheimer's fall asleep in front of the TV and/or spend hours in front of it. We chose not to do that. The American Academy of Pediatrics recommends no TV time for children under two and then only limited time after that. I think that's a good rule of thumb for Alzheimer's couples too.

- Our lullaby music—*Songs of Innocence (Lullabies for Us All)*—work their magic for adults as well as children. You can order them on Amazon.com.

- For more about Mike's changing sleep patterns in the final months, check the tips in Chapter 50 (Keeping our Marriage Bed).

PART VII

~

Still Savoring Life
at Year 5

CHAPTER 29

WHAT LIFE WAS LIKE FOR
MIKE AND ME IN YEAR 5

*In this chapter my journal notes
recall some surprising good news
from the halfway point of
our journey.*

THERE ARE LOTS OF SCARY STORIES ABOUT ALZHEIMER'S,
so it's not surprising that Alzheimer's couples wonder and worry
about the terrible things that might happen as the disease progresses.

I know I started worrying as soon as Mike was diagnosed: When
will Mike stop knowing who I am? When will he no longer love me
or our children? How fast will his coordination and physical skills
decline? Will there come a time when he will start wandering out of
the house or getting lost?

And perhaps the scariest of all—when will his disposition start
turning to the rage or aggression often associated with Alzheimer's?

Since every couple is different—and every Alzheimer's patient
responds in his or her own way to the disease—there is really no
way to predict exactly what your journey will hold. But I can tell you
that there is no reason for you and your partner to automatically
expect the worst.

Despite all the problems that Alzheimer's brought to Mike and
me, we still discovered that each year held pleasant surprises and
reasons for joy. To help dramatize this for you and your loved one,
I have used my journal entries in this chapter to provide you with a
running account of what Mike and I experienced in year five—the

halfway point of our nearly 10-year Alzheimer's journey.

I think these particular journal entries bring to light several surprising and hopeful points:

1. Mike still knew me and loved me at the halfway point, and I still loved him more than ever.

2. Mike was not an angry person in year five. In fact, we had no more concerns about anger than in years past.

3. Mike's physical and mental skills were indeed diminishing over time, but my journal entries show that we were successfully adjusting and continuing our relationship together.

Most important of all, the following excerpts from my Year 5 journal show that, despite Alzheimer's, life does go on—it *must* go on—with all its ups and downs, laughter, love, tears and celebrations.

It may sound trite, but a positive attitude can play such an important role in the quality of your Alzheimer's journey. After Mike was diagnosed, it took a while, but he and I eventually resolved to place our focus on the rest of his life, rather than the end of his life. I believe this attitude we adopted—this choice to keep our relationship alive and to live each day to the fullest—allowed us to stay active and in touch, long after the typical Alzheimer's projections suggested otherwise.

Now, I invite you to sit back and get to know what the world was like for Mike and me 5 years after he was first diagnosed.

⤙ FROM MY JOURNAL ⤚

JANUARY (YEAR 5)
MIKE CONTINUES TO MAKE ME LAUGH...

Mike and I took a few days and went to Cannon Beach. On Tuesday night we went to Mt. St. Helens, Wednesday stayed at Stephanie Inn, and Thursday at Aberdeen. Stephanie Inn is wonderful, walked into town and enjoyed a romantic slow start to our day. Loved the excellent breakfast and reading One for the Money *as*

*we looked out at the waves. We departed our hotel at 11:58 a.m.
having enjoyed every minute before our checkout time at noon.*

~

*Mike continues to laugh and make me happy. When heading into
St. Helens we saw lots of country life: old buildings, cars, country
store and those new little Mini Coopers that made us laugh. We felt
like we were really out and away from everything.*

~

*Last night we watched "Oprah." The show triggered some past sad
memories in our relationship. Mike came and sat on the couch with
me... putting his arm around me, giving me kisses, and telling me
he loves me. I am so lucky Mike can still say and feel these things.*

~

*Last time Mike drove was when he brought the Subaru home from
the repair shop. His not driving has relieved a big worry for me.
So nice Mike can still say he is sorry when he is grouchy.*

FEBRUARY (YEAR 5)

MIKE AND I CELEBRATE VALENTINE'S DAY...

*Mike and I had a lovely Valentine's Day together. We drove to
Hallmark in Poulsbo on the 13th, and Mike bought cards while I
waited in the car. He later showed me Kathleen's cards—they are
lovely. When I told him how nice they were, he said, "I mean it."
He really had to work at signing them before
we went to her apartment.*

*Mike and I went to Seattle for Valentine's Day, it is so good to
make the effort! On our ride to the 8:45 a.m. ferry Mike said,
"This is fun, I haven't done this in a long time."*

~

Breakfast at Pike Place Market, stopped at See's Candies, bought shoes at The Walking Company, and wonderful French bakery shop for lunch and special dinner dessert.

Mike forgot to bring my Valentine's Day card… he left it on the table because he couldn't get it in the envelope—it was unsigned. I may ask him to sign it today. It may be the last card he is able to sign for me.

~

I continue to do most of the talking, but Mike is congenial and good company.

I'm feeling sad as I write. Mike couldn't follow my discussion of bringing in the wood from the front porch. He said he couldn't see it in his mind. I need to remember to show him what I want done. He cannot see it in his mind when I say it. I am so glad he can still tell me these things.

~

Mike likes to help me cook. Eating is becoming more difficult for him… he went to get a knife, came back with a fork, two knives, and two spoons. Sometimes he doesn't get enough to eat. He doesn't think about time and when he should eat.

~

Reading together is lovely, he can help me with words I don't know while I read out loud.

~

I had coffee with a friend and she suggested a support group for me. Maybe it is time I go, but right now life is good! Time to go back for a quick snuggle with Mike before I get ready to take a walk with Wendy.

MORE CHANGES IN MIKE'S ABILITIES...

Friday was a difficult day with Mike. He was angry over not driving, so we called to set up a driving test for him. Short with me when I said we could get more corduroy slacks in Victoria. He said we could get them on the internet. I told him he was unnecessarily grouchy. When I came to bed he said he was sorry.

~

Enjoyed talking to a New Mom's group in Ballard, while Mike hung out with Pat. Later we all enjoyed an Italian dinner together. Saturday Kathleen and Sam hung out with Mike all day while I taught the Couples' Relationship class at Swedish. I am so lucky to have both Patrick and Kathleen in my life.

~

Some of Mike's quotes I want to remember:
- *"You have no idea how frustrating it is."*
- *"I know what I want to say."*
- *"It is all up there."*
- *"What I want to do is figure out how to talk."*

~

Tea at the Poulsbo Bakery with the newspaper is a perfect break for me!!!

~

Mike and I went to see the movie Eight Below. When I asked how he would rate it he said, "Sweet." Had Indian food at the Pavilion, then hot tub at home, and read the third Evanovich book in bed.

~

We had dinner at Bill and Candy's. When I asked Mike how it was for him, he said "Fun." When I asked about his ability to interact, he said, "It is what it is." We both had a fun night with lots of laughter.

~

I need things to look forward to. Must remember to keep mak-
ing outings: Alaska in August . . . Trip to Vancouver Island in
VW camper . . . A water well put in at Mt. Brook

MAY (YEAR 5)

I FREQUENTLY TELL MIKE I LOVE HIM...

Patrick calls often and continues to be a listening ear. Yesterday I
told him how difficult it was moving a desk with his dad who could
not figure out left, right, up or down. Patrick listened to my story
then said, "How are you?"

(Note to reader: I was talking about Mike but Patrick thought
to ask about me. From the east coast he was providing a great
deal of care and support for his mom.)

~

Kathleen's 32nd birthday was fun. Went shopping at the mall,
then Thai food at the house with Sam and Mike. She is like a ray
of sunshine—pretty, happy, fun, and so willing to help.

~

Kathleen asked if I found it difficult to deal with Alzheimer's when
with other people. I told her about Michael Douglas and how he
was not embarrassed by his dad (Kirk Douglas), even when Kirk
had trouble speaking on national television. I told her I want to be
like Michael Douglas and enjoy Mike for who he is.

~

Mike is so patient over loss of speech. Difficult to get complete
thought, but we usually figure it out.

~

I need to listen to Mike's clear suggestions. Most recently, he was so
gentle when he told me, "We need to be careful in what we put in
the garbage. We do a good job, but could be better."

I frequently tell Mike I love him. He says "why?" I need to be more specific about what he does for me!

~

When I went to bed last night, I was feeling sad thinking about how Mike is doing less than before and I cannot change the course. I shared the thought with him and feel better this morning.

~

Wonderful Mother's Day. Kathleen did so many nice things; she keeps my cup full. Always there when I need her which is increasing. We had a family BBQ on the deck with family and friends, thirteen people in all and it worked.

~

It might be helpful to continue talking to Mike about my emotions even when he cannot fully understand.

~

Increased problem with clothing: slacks, belt, jacket, and shoes. More problems taking pills on his own.

~

I read a little of the Customs Newsletter to Mike and asked if there was a part he wanted read. He said, "I like it all." We put it by the couch so I can read it all to him. Nice to go to bed at the same time and snuggle.

JULY (YEAR 5)
I NEED TO LET MIKE BE MIKE...

Yesterday Patrick, Kathleen, and I saw Dr. Jung without Mike. What we learned:

- *In six months, need to have continual care to keep Mike safe.*
- *I should probably not leave Mike alone now.*
- *May need to take away car keys, put locks on doors, safety bars, have assistance 2-3 nights a week so I can sleep.*

- Need to find backup, someone to help when family not available and I have to work.
- Dr. Jung does not think Mike will be aggressive.
- Medication is clearly not helping as much as it had.

Lots to think about emotionally. Both Kathleen and Patrick were exceptionally good with asking questions. I am so lucky to have them.

~

Hot trip home from Montana. We stopped at Moses Lake Park. While I took a little nap in the VW camper, Mike found a stand with snow cones and brought two back to the camper. It was like a dream to see him with snow cones in his hands when I awoke.

~

Kathleen says, "Dad loves you so much; he wants to do things for you." I need to remember to let Mike be Mike. We like to play music and dance together.

~

Mike put his arms around me in the kitchen today and said, "Did I tell you how much I love you?" I told him "Not today" and got a big hug from him. Mike continues to give love.

~

Woke up to a story on NPR about seniors getting swindled. Mike's first words were, "We have to get in on that."
We laughed and laughed!

SEPTEMBER (YEAR 5)
LIFE IS GOOD…

I am surprised it has been so long since I have written. I think that is a sign that life is good or life is busy.

~

We had a wonderful trip to Alaska, fun sister time for me,

and special moments with Mike. It was a special time for us at
Chena Hot Springs in our little cabin.

~

Went with Stan and Audrey for pizza. Audrey said that she and
Stan talked about it and they want Mike to come over one day a
week. What a wonderful offer and just what we need.
We are so lucky to have good friends in our life.

~

Mike got angry over the doctor who told him not to drive. "I never
should have gone," he said. Then he said, "No point in being mad."

~

We are talking about going to Mt. Brook to put in a well—
another good time!

~

Reminder: get Victor Borge DVD. Mike likes his humor.

~

Mike now has trouble with spaces. Sitting on chairs, pulling them
out and maneuvering around table legs, walking between groups
of people. Frequently goes in the wrong direction in the house. But
gets things done if he has enough time and I leave him alone.

~

Mike is with Stan and I miss him. I am off to teach at
Swedish Hospital.

~

Nice working in the yard and on the deck with Mike the past two
days. As Mike gets more dependent, I am finding it difficult to leave
him. Why? Maybe just knowing he is vulnerable, and not knowing
how long we have. I love him so very much.

OCTOBER (YEAR 5)
MIKE CONTINUES TO AMAZE ME...

Start of a wonderful trip with Kathleen and Sam to Mt. Brook. So many touching memories, but the best one: Kathleen and Sam got engaged! Mike was so pleased. He said, "You're going to make me cry... this is a new chapter... Yippee."

~

Mike continues to amaze me, his laughter and good humor make necessary changes easy.

One day on our way into town from the cabin he said he wanted a gate to block the lower road. I was happy with all the projects we had done and said, "We did the water witcher, a well, the insulation, and the road to the well. And now you want a gate!" Mike began to tear up. When I asked him why he said, "Because I want to do all those things for you."

We pulled off the dirt road to talk. I said I could be married to a lot of people who could do those things, but not care if they did them for me. Your gift is that you want to do them for me. Mike cried and we hugged. I am so lucky to still have the emotional Mike I love.

~

Mike is so happy that Sam will be part of our family. My hope is that Mike is still well in July or August for the wedding. Either way we know he enjoyed the moment of knowing Kathleen will be married to Sam. The good news is that Mike continues to think about things. Most of his clear thoughts are midday.

~

We are doing surprisingly well at Mt. Brook. Outings and interactions with others are helpful: neighbors, church, and also having Kathleen and Sam joining us.

~

Sometimes I am not patient, I need to write when I feel that way and not take it out on Mike.

~

Mike likes to wander around the cabin nude—nothing new. Gets ready for bed and forgets something. Last night it was his mouth guard. I am brushing my teeth and in he walks. I was a little grouchy: "I thought you were ready for bed but you're walking around with no clothes on." It makes me smile now when I think about it.

~

Mike has been dreaming and recalling old memories. He awakened one morning and said, "I dreamed about George" (his stepdad). "I should have been nicer to him."

~

Mike and I do well at Mt. Brook, such simple days: Mike chops wood, we eat, and I read aloud. The Janet Evanovich books are great for us. We are on book ten, got it from Mt. Brook Library.

~

I continue to enjoy my emotional and physical connection with Mike. It is nice he is still able to give both. I love his, "Good night, Sweetheart." And when I say, "I love you" he says, "I know you do."

~

Another recent change for Mike: The words, "up, down, over, under" are now all confusing for him.

~

I cannot sleep—thinking, "What will I do when Mike cannot care for himself with body functions?"

NOVEMBER (YEAR 5)
MIKE HAS DECIDED NOT TO LET THIS GET TO HIM...

Mike saw Dr. Jung in Seattle today. She is such a perfect doctor for him and me! He tested better this time, amazing! When asked how he was doing, he said, "I decided not to let this get to me."

Results of Dr. Jung's testing:
- *Mike continues to be able to recall three things after a time lapse. Jung told him absolutely amazing! "You can do this because you are smart and have lots of wiring. You are able to go around (a topic) and get to it a different way."*
- *Mike kept working at a complicated drawing in Dr. Jung's office until he got a little angry but just pushed harder and got closer to doing it.*
- *Dr. Jung said, "You're a smart cookie." Mike liked that.*

On our way to Stan's, Mike said, "I just wish I could talk."

~

Christmas was perfect. (I wrote a number of pages about wonderful memories of the holiday with Mike, family and friends, including way too much food!)

Christmas gifts for Mike:
- *Slip-on shoes: watching Pat help put them on Mike made me laugh.*
- *Sweater: Kathleen's turn to help Mike, another smile for me.*
- *Electric Shaver: watching Pat help his dad shave—more smiles.*

(continued next page)
(Note to reader: I also remember some tears at this time as we all felt this would be the last Christmas Mike would be fully present. But we did have fun. What a special holiday!)

~

New developments with Mike:
- *gets confused about what things are garbage*
- *goes to do something and forgets while en route*
- *dressing is difficult, getting arms in sleeves, etc.*
- *speech is getting much more challenging; Mike does a great job of not getting upset and continuing to work at it.*

INSIGHTS

- Reading my journal notes reminds me what special moments we still had together in the fifth year after diagnosis.

- Yes, we were still in love, could go to Montana, have fun experiences with our children, celebrate the joy of a future wedding in our family, and had figured out how to adjust to the changes that were going on around us.

- Now that you know Mike and I were still very much in love at this point in the illness, my hope is that you, too, can stay in love—or fall in love all over again—even as the disease progresses.

- It is clear that Mike had moments of being angry like we all do, but he was not a threat to me, himself, or others, and Dr. Jung said that anger would not necessarily be a problem.

- The new challenges were Mike's speech, which was getting more difficult to understand, his physical needs, which were increasing, and his dwindling independence (he could no longer be left alone). Each had an increasing impact on us and those around us.

- Mike's positive attitude was still present at Year 5 and made a difference in each and every day. I believe that attitude is a choice we make about how we decide to deal with whatever comes our way in life. Mike and I chose to deal with Alzheimer's by being positive instead of negative and living each day to the fullest. I'm sure that choosing a positive attitude allowed us to stay active and in touch with each other for years longer than expected.

- In Year 5 we were still a couple, and still experiencing all the ups and downs of typical couples. There were moments of laughter and joy, as well as times we were short with each other. This "normalcy" is something every Alzheimer's couple should strive for as long as possible.

- Remember: Just because the end of life may seem more imminent with Alzheimer's, don't let that distract you and your partner from all the rich, beautiful life that still remains in the middle and later stages of this disease.

- "Every day can be a miniature life for those who are fully present," wrote Emerson. Mike and I definitely discovered the truth in that.

CHAPTER 30

WHEN MIKE COULD NO LONGER BE LEFT ALONE

*Would this new development
threaten our stay-at-home plan?*

TOWARD THE END OF THE FIFTH YEAR OF MIKE'S ILLNESS, a new urgency came into our lives. Noting how Mike's abilities were declining, Dr. Jung alerted us that he should no longer be left alone. Within six months we needed to have things in place so Mike would have continual 24/7 care to keep him safe.

That news was life-altering for both of us. Mike was an independent guy who liked to do his own thing. I knew he would not go down without a fight on this one, and I wondered how well I would manage this new challenge.

I also wondered how well I could manage being with Mike (or anyone else for that matter) all day every day. As the disease progressed, I willingly took over more and more of the everyday responsibilities. For example, I was now the driver when we went places together, but I could still leave Mike alone at home if I needed to make a quick run for groceries or a stop at the bank. Now, there would be no more of that, and so many other everyday things. Yes, being together 24/7 would be a real challenge and, quite honestly, I wasn't sure how I would adapt to it.

With this new change that was rushing at us, we clearly needed to reach out for more help. I felt that friends and family were already giving all that they could. Asking them to do even more, so Mike would never be alone—well, I felt that I just couldn't do that for they, too, had lives of their own.

We had come to the point where it was now necessary to consider professional caregivers, or maybe even adult daycare centers.

WOULD MIKE GO ALONG WITH THE PLAN?

First, of course, I had to get Mike to go along with the whole idea of 24/7 care, which I suspected would be no easy matter. He did not like the idea of including other people in our lives when he was so vulnerable. Besides, he was not convinced that it was even necessary to have someone stay with him. So his first reaction was to inform me that he could stay by himself or with his friend Stan.

At that point I could have given Mike a big list of reasons why he could no longer stay safely by himself: forgets to eat, doesn't take his medication, might leave the stove on, doesn't always answer the phone when I call, and the list goes on.

Instead, I reminded him that I was on his side and we needed to work together on this new phase. If Dr. Jung said 24/7 care was necessary, then I needed him to willingly agree to do this for me.

I reminded him of the original deal we had agreed on, five years before—that by working together, we could avoid moving him to a care facility. He was going to stay at home with me, but in order for that to happen, I needed some breaks in my daily schedule, and I needed his cooperation to make that happen.

Mike wanted to help me in any way he could so asking him to do this for me was pretty compelling and gave him a reason to want to go along with the new plan. He got it, and agreed. Once again, we had talked it through as husband and wife and were on the same page together. From there I started exploring options, starting with daycare.

INVESTIGATING ADULT DAYCARE

I had heard about a couple of daycare options for adults not far from our home and thought that would be a good place to start. Because Mike and I were a team and this was to be an important decision, we went to look at the daycare facilities together.

We first visited a center for adults with limited abilities, both physical and mental. It was just fifteen minutes from our home and I was impressed with the range of activities. Unfortunately, these activities were not ones that Mike would be able to participate in. And the individuals who attended were not in Mike's age group and did not have Alzheimer's. That facility was not a match for us.

Next we scheduled a tour of a facility twenty minutes from us that offered both adult daycare and long-term care. They not only gave us a tour but provided lunch while we talked with the nurse manager and social worker. It was all very pleasant.

Later Mike and I talked at length about the facility. They offered a $10/hour adult daycare option, or a full weekend stay for only $100. It seemed like just what we needed. It would provide a break for me and be a safe place for Mike. However, Mike was not buying it!

We had multiple conversations and I finally convinced Mike to try spending a few hours at the facility; this was something he could do for me. I reminded him again that we had a plan; he would stay at home with me but, for this to happen, I needed to have a way to go to work and have time away now and then. So we decided to give it a try—a practice day—only 2–3 hours as I recall. Mike would go to the daycare facility in the morning, and I would pick him up after lunch.

When I returned to pick him up, Mike was sitting by the large flat-screen TV with a program on he did not like and pie scattered all about—in his lap and on the floor.

I signed Mike out, and asked him about his day. With his limited speech he said, "They took me a ride." He pointed out the window, indicating that they had ridden along the water, the same way we were driving. I said, "That was nice," but he shook his head and frowned. It seemed that it was all sort of silly to him as he rode this way all the time. Oh well, it would not be something we would do again.

Because we live on an island, our daycare choices were limited. While we did not find a good nearby adult daycare center for Mike, you will probably have better luck if you live in a more populated area. I know there are excellent options in many communities.

As for me, I now wondered, "If daycare is not a good option for Mike and me, what should we do next?" Fortunately, Dr. Jung had given us a six-month window to come up with a solution for 24/7 care, so I was still optimistic.

In the back of my mind, though, I worried that I would soon have to give up my work in order to provide Mike with the added care he now needed. I was willing to do that, if necessary. But teaching parent education classes was not only rewarding for me, it also gave me a needed break away from Mike and our life with Alzheimer's. I had hoped to continue teaching the Lamaze Getaway Workshop and classes at the Swedish Medical Center, but now wondered if that would be possible.

It was at that critical point that a family friend named Stephanie came into our lives and changed everything for the better (see the next chapter for her story).

INSIGHTS

- I learned something very important while searching for an adult daycare. I learned that I needed to keep Mike on the team, for without his help everything would have been much harder. I just had to remember to slow down and let him know exactly what he could do for me and for us, and why. If I clearly and patiently explained things, he was there for me, for he wanted to help me in any way he could.

- It was also important for me to remember that Mike, like everyone, wanted to feel valued and useful. By reminding him that I really did need his help, I provided that opportunity for him.

- This process made me think of mothers when they go back to work and the challenge they face to find the right daycare option for their child. While Mike was certainly not a child, it was the same because I was entrusting someone I did not know to care for my husband.

- Good facilities that offer adult day care are not always easy to find, nor is it easy to find people who are a good fit for you and your family in your home, but it is possible. Just hang in there, knowing there is the right kind of help out there for the persistent.

CHAPTER 31

HIRING A FAMILY FRIEND TO HELP

When, why and how we found and hired an angel named Stephanie.

OUR SEARCH FOR A GOOD local adult daycare had not worked out, but we still needed some sort of part-time help for Mike and me at this midpoint of Mike's illness.

At this stage, Mike did not require a professional caregiver (that would come a few years later with Sabina). For now, he just needed a caring person who could keep him company while I was away at work, make sure he was safe, that his medications were taken on time, that he had healthy meals and an occasional outing to chase away boredom.

At first Mike continued to resist the idea of having an outsider stay with him in our home; he still felt he could take care of himself. Fortunately, our daughter had an idea that seemed to be acceptable to everyone: She suggested that her friend Stephanie might be able to help part-time on the days I worked and perhaps other times too.

Mike and I both knew and liked Stephanie, so it was not difficult to convince Mike to go along with her giving him a hand. But I wondered if she would be willing to enter the world of Alzheimer's with us. Fortunately, she was!

THE RIGHT PERSON AT THE RIGHT TIME

Stephanie was not a professional caregiver, but she was a quality person, a wife and mother, and someone who knew and cared about our family. She had a gentle manner, a friendly smile and a ready laugh. She was always willing to try anything with Mike and if it didn't work out that was okay—she was more than willing to try a different plan next time. And what I appreciated most of all was that she could be sensitive to Mike's emotions and mood swings which turned out to be more and more important as the disease progressed.

Whenever Stephanie came to our house, new energy came into our home. At first she did just what we asked, provided company for Mike, made sure pills were taken and a meal prepared; later she did far more than I ever expected and helped in virtually all of Mike's daily care.

Stephanie lightened the load for me in so many ways. When I was out of town teaching a Getaway Weekend class, she became part of our family team that would come and care for Mike for an entire weekend. But she was also happy to be my readily available "fill-in" person, allowing me to step away for a few hours for my book club or support group, both of which were important to me. And, in the last six months or so whenever our granddaughter was with us for the day, Stephanie was there to ensure that I did not have to be vigilant of Mike's every need throughout the day.

I remember fondly the days when Stephanie arrived with a smile, always ready for anything we had scheduled. She would help me get Mike up and out of bed and then, if he was up for it (and he usually was), they would go for a car ride.

I loved to see them off on their little outings. Stephanie would usually give Mike a stick of gum and turn on his favorite Anne Murray CD—and then off they would go for the day's adventure. As I waved to them, I could actually feel my shoulders relax and I would breathe a little easier. Clearly, Stephanie's presence was not only good for Mike, it was good for me too.

When they returned, Stephanie and I prepared lunch, which we typically enjoyed on the outdoor deck before we settled Mike for his afternoon nap. Then Stephanie was out the door and on to her own life of children, husband and more. As for Mike and me, thanks to Stephanie and the all-important break she provided us, we could continue the rest of our day, feeling a little more patient and loving toward each other.

So for now, it turned out that we did not need a daycare facility for Mike, nor did he need to live in a care facility or have a professional in-house caregiver. Instead, we could continue to live fairly independently in our own home because we now had an angel named Stephanie in our life.

INSIGHTS

- Be aware that the middle years of this disease might send you a false signal that you and your loved one can no longer deal with Alzheimer's together in your home. As things become more difficult, you may think that you need to turn to an outside care facility or a full-time professional caregiver when all you may really need is a little help from a caring part-time person.

- When the time comes, it's my hope that you will be fortunate enough to look around and discover someone like Stephanie in your world; someone who is a natural caregiver and helper; someone with a big heart and a sunny disposition who innately understands your journey with Alzheimer's and is willing to lend a helping hand.

- I've learned that natural caregivers like Stephanie can teach us so much. Among other things, Stephanie taught me to keep smiling and laughing, to take a deep breath now and then, to look after myself as well as Mike, and to ask for help whenever I needed it.

- In the long run, building a circle of friends, family, and professionals who can help you is the only practical way you and your loved one can continue to live with Alzheimer's at home. You can do this together with your loved one, but you have to have help to ensure that Alzheimer's doesn't become more than you can manage.

- Stephanie is one of the very important people who made it possible for me to be not just Mike's caregiver, but to continue being his loving wife.

CHAPTER 32

CAN A SPOUSE BE A CAREGIVER AND STILL BE A SPOUSE?

Balancing the two roles may be tricky but, with intention and planning, it can definitely be done.

EARLY IN MIKE'S ILLNESS A FRIEND CAUTIONED ME that I would have to make a difficult choice: I could either choose to be a good wife or a good caregiver—but I couldn't really choose both. She said the demands of filling both roles would eventually become too much.

Some time later another friend who had taken care of her husband in their home at the end of his life told me, "I only wish I could have been more of a wife than a caregiver for him."

There it was again. I did not want to have that regret. When Mike was first diagnosed with Alzheimer's we had agreed that he was going to live at home; and we had also committed to continue nurturing our marriage and our love story, for better or worse, in sickness and in health.

At first I couldn't imagine how our marriage would ever be in jeopardy. But starting in year five, when Mike could no longer be left alone, things began to change. I could see that being together 24/7 put a new kind of stress on our relationship. I loved Mike dearly and wanted to stay in love with him, but if all I did was his physical care and there was no time left for us or our relationship, that could change everything.

Despite the earlier warnings from my friends (or perhaps because of them), it turned out to be relatively easy to be both a caregiver and wife as long as I did two things: The first was to take good care of my relationship with Mike, and the second was to take good care of me.

TAKING GOOD CARE OF OUR RELATIONSHIP

For years I had been teaching the Gottman "new parent relationship" classes. It turned out that some of the principles from that class became guiding lights for Mike and me on our Alzheimer's journey. Here are some of the simple practices that helped keep our marriage alive and healthy:

- Mike and I kept our daily conversations going. Even when Mike could no longer express himself very well, we made time to talk and I helped fill in the words for him.

- We made a daily ritual of departures and reunions. If I left the house, I would always pause to give him a kiss goodbye, and I always greeted him when I returned. I would talk to the care provider too, but only after I warmly greeted Mike.

- I praised him for what he did right, rather than focus on what he did wrong.

- We took time to reminisce about our lifelong love story.

- We found joy and humor in every day, laughing about the funny little things that happened.

- We continued to create love stories by going places together and experiencing life as a couple.

- I was patient with Mike and was careful not to criticize him, especially when we were with others.

- I listened to him and showed that I sincerely valued what he had to say, even when his cognitive abilities continued to decline because of Alzheimer's.

Mike did his part, too, by thanking me, flirting with me, giving me kisses or a smile, and letting me know that I, too, was appreciated, which made it all so worthwhile.

TAKING GOOD CARE OF MYSELF

Everyone needs breaks in their routine but this is especially true of caregivers. Our family and friends had made it possible for me to continue my work outside our home and to have little breaks away from Mike. But I soon learned that, if I was going to remain both a loving wife and a full-time caregiver, I was going to need more time away. When I did not take care of me I would become irritable, short-tempered, and exhausted—and that led to everything else becoming frayed.

So here are the gems that worked for me:

- I learned to snatch and enjoy quiet moments of solitude every day, either in the morning before Mike got up or after he went to bed.

- I found quiet time to journal; it allowed me to process what was happening in my life and what I was feeling.

- A hot bath at the end of the day was a perfect way for me to pamper myself and settle in for the night.

- I took catnaps and slept when Mike slept.

- I scheduled time away, not just a few hours but a complete night or two when I could.

- I enjoyed walks in the neighborhood, on the beach, or up the long hill to Swedish Hospital when I walked to work after my ferry ride. (If walking isn't your first choice, take a yoga or exercise class.)

- I learned to grab a nice quiet meal out by myself.

- I gave myself permission to allow friends and family to give me breaks here and there.

- I learned NOT to give up special moments with friends, including birthday outings, book club meetings, or walks and talks.
- I continued to work because my job was an important part of being me.

Mike did his part here, too, for he never questioned my time away. He wanted me to have fun without feeling guilty, and enjoyed my coming home with a smile on my face and some stories to share.

So here is what I now know: Be assured that you really *can* be both a loving spouse and a great caregiver for your loved one—but you cannot do it alone. You need help from your friends, family, and professionals too. With their help here and there, you can take good care of your relationship, while also taking care of you. So give yourself a break now and then, and hold on to who you are. Taking care of yourself is essential to taking care of the one you love.

CHAPTER 33

GOOD REASONS TO JOIN
A SUPPORT GROUP

---

*By year 5, I knew I needed to be with
people who truly understood what it's
like to care for someone 24/7.*

EARLIER IN THE BOOK, I URGED YOU to create your circle of friends and family. It's my belief that your inner circle can make it possible for you and your loved one to continue living your lives together at home despite the disease. Now I urge every caregiver who reads these words to also join a support group. Hopefully my own experience with this option will show you why.

Midway in Mike's disease various people started telling me that I should attend a support group. While it sounded like reasonable advice, I could always find good reasons to ignore it, including: I was hesitant to talk with strangers about my problems. I was reluctant to share my inner feelings and sadness with others. And I definitely didn't want to talk about Mike "behind his back."

Besides, there was also the problem of the location and time of day, and who could stay with Mike while I was with my support group. It all seemed overwhelming, so I just put it off as long as possible.

As time went on, and caring for Mike became more difficult, I realized that I simply had to have a safe place to vent. I knew I needed to be with people who truly understood what this was all about—what it's like to care for someone 24/7. Now I was ready for a support group, but was there a good group that was ready for me?

FINDING THE RIGHT SUPPORT GROUP FOR YOU

Ideally, the Alzheimer's Association can help you find a nearby support group that specializes in Alzheimer's and meets at convenient times for you. (See the Insights section below).

If you can't find an Alzheimer's group, look for one that welcomes all caregivers. Since I live on an island, that's what I did, and it worked out great.

Our little group met on Tuesdays from 2:00 to 3:30 and varied in size from 2 or 3 members to as many as 12 or 13. That was part of the beauty of the group—go when you can, always welcome but never obligated.

Some of us were dealing with Alzheimer's, but others were dealing with cancer, stroke or other conditions. While the diseases were different, I learned quickly that the feelings, concerns and fears that all caregivers face are virtually the same.

Karen our group leader was always there with a warm welcome and listening heart. She was our guide—never telling us what to do or how to feel; always guiding us to our own discoveries; giving each person time to share or not share as they wish; watching the time for us; balancing each individual's needs; and updating us about those who could not attend that day.

And, most important, Karen made it possible for us to share our feelings, hopes and worries in a confidential and non-judgmental setting.

WHAT A SUPPORT GROUP GIVES YOU

Karen's support group gave me priceless gifts and insights that I did not expect but still appreciate to this day, including:

- The peace of mind in knowing that Mike and I were not alone and that others shared similar frustrations and problems.
- The relief of being able to share my honest feelings when I was sad, overwhelmed, or angry.

- The comfort of knowing that I could cry and laugh in a safe space.
- A greater understanding of the emotional and financial toll of providing home care for another.
- The ability to listen to (and care about) the sadness of others without taking it on.
- The satisfaction of sharing my personal Alzheimer's experience in a way that could help others.
- A greater awareness of the many resources available in our community.
- The gift of meeting caring men and women who are still my friends today.

--- **INSIGHTS** ---

- The Alzheimer's Association can help you locate a Support Group in your area. Just search Alzheimer's Association Support Groups for Caregivers and then click on your state.
- Alzheimer's care facilities often provide support groups that welcome anyone who would like to attend.
- If you discover you can't always attend a support group in person, the Alzheimer's Association web page lists "online" support groups, both for caregivers and for those who have the disease.
- My community on Bainbridge Island sponsors a group called Island Volunteer Caregivers, which has a support group component. Thankfully I found this wonderful resource. Search carefully and you might find something similar at a church or social center in your community.
- Remember that caring, courage and compassion are what you receive in a support group, but you have the honor of giving them as well.
- Two helpful rules of thumb for participation in a support group from Karen, my group leader: 1. Listen with the intent to understand, not to reply. 2. Listen with your heart, not your voice or your head.

PART VIII

~

Keeping Up With Our Children
and Grandchildren

CHAPTER 34

CELEBRATING OUR DAUGHTER'S WEDDING

*The day your child marries is one of
life's most treasured events.*

IT WAS AUGUST, six-and-a-half years after Mike was diagnosed, and we were both excited. This was the month our daughter Kathleen would be married to Sam.

Ten months earlier, when Kathleen and Sam had announced their engagement, Mike had asked, "What can I do?" I told him he would have the important job of walking our daughter down the aisle and "giving her away." I was quite sure he understood the honor, but I now wondered if Mike could actually pull it off.

During the months leading up to the wedding, Mike's memory, balance and mobility had continued to decline. He was still walking, but his ability to sit down had become a challenge, for he had trouble finding the chair. When he sat, I needed to be vigilant, always ready to pull a chair under him or push him a little to the right or left so he did not miss his landing spot.

He and I were still able to communicate, but he could no longer commit a line to memory and then deliver it at the proper time. I thought of a way to solve that problem, and I was pretty sure he could walk Kathleen down the aisle, but I worried about him missing the chair when he attempted to sit down.

The day your child marries is one of life's most treasured events—something to be anticipated, celebrated and remembered. I knew Mike would not always be able to remember the day but, for now, he was definitely enjoying the moment. Our little strawberry-blond baby girl would be marrying Sam, and Mike and I could not have been more pleased to have Sam join our family.

There are lots of hard times with Alzheimer's, and some that are easier, and then there are certain times when you just need to sit back and savor the moment together. This was one of those times.

Kathleen and Sam were to be married in a peaceful garden, at a farm, just a short 20-minute drive from our home on Bainbridge Island. The setting would be pastoral and beautiful.

Mike wanted to know what Sam would be wearing. Kathleen explained that Sam would be wearing a tux, and then went on to tell her dad that it wasn't necessary for him to wear one. Well, when Mike found out that Sam would be wearing a tux, he insisted on wearing one too. Going to the rental place and getting Mike fitted was a little tricky, but we managed. And Mike was delighted with his formal look.

As with all the best celebrations, people come from afar and it is a time to catch up with old friends and share fond memories. Kathleen and Sam's wedding was all of that. Our home was filled with family who were staying over, and with friends who were staying in nearby motels or B&Bs.

Mike liked all the activity, and it was surprisingly easy for me because all these people loved Mike. They were happy to slide that chair under him and they brought him lots of hugs, laughter and stories of times gone by. My tasks were relatively easy: keep Mike's schedule the same, meals and medication on time, and never forget the crucial afternoon nap.

OKAY, HERE WE GO

I have so many fond memories of that day. One of the sweetest is the image of Harry, my sister's husband, tying Mike's fancy tux tie, while Mike hammed it up. Mike looked very cute! Perhaps some would say handsome, but he was short and the tux a little large, so "cute" is the word I use with love for the man I had wed some 41 years before.

There were a lot of little things going on for Mike that day—stand here for photos, sit over there, wait here, I'll be right back—but finally it was time for the all-important walk down the aisle. I took a deep breath and thought, "Okay, here we go."

Kathleen and her dad took their appointed place in a little stand of trees, well beyond the folding chairs on the lawn and out of sight of the guests. With tears in my eyes I took my walk down the formal path, arm-in-arm with one of Sam's dear friends. Then I sat and turned in anticipation of our daughter's walk with her dad. I could see them standing together and Mike giving Kathleen a kiss on the cheek; I wondered again, how will this part of the wedding go?

Now a friend softly played a guitar and our beautiful daughter and her dad began their walk down the garden path together. (More tears and silent thoughts: you are doing great honey, keep up the good work.) There was no fancy footwork that day, but the walk was successfully completed and Mike's mission accomplished.

And now it was time for the words. At this point, I joined Mike and stood with him and Kathleen, and when asked, "Who gives this woman away?" I said, "We do."

One last challenge, now. It was time for Mike to turn and sit. The first turn went well, and then the other turn. There was no folding chair awaiting us, for we had set up a nice wide bench with a back and arms on the side. When Mike began to sit with his arm on the armrest, I was ready and gave the crucial little push and he landed. No one applauded for Mike, but I'm quite sure there were several friends and family members that day who wanted to. Yes, Mike was able to do his part for Kathleen on her special day. From there, Mike and I settled in together, sitting close, holding hands, and enjoying every moment. I could feel the presence of friends and family, as two happy young people made a lifetime commitment to each other, "For better, or worse, in sickness and in health, until death do us part." Kathleen and Sam were making their commitment, and Mike and I were living ours.

The reception was fun and easy. I made our toast to the bride and groom as Mike looked on approvingly. Then he danced with his daughter and with me. I was not "on duty" that night with Mike, because Patrick, family, and friends were all there for him too. It was a night to remember with laughter and tears. The tears were of joy, of course, because I knew this was a moment in our lives like no other.

I still don't know all the little backstories of what it was like for our daughter having a dad with Alzheimer's while planning the most important event of her life. Mike was such an unknown for her special day, and yet there was never a question in Kathleen's mind that her dad would not only be there, but he would be a real part of her celebration.

I wondered what was said between father and daughter before they walked down the garden path. Did he give her words of advice, tell her she was cherished, remind her how beautiful she was that day, and that we were so happy for her? I didn't think so.

Years later, Kathleen told me what her dad actually said that day. He said, "What do we do now?"

She just smiled and responded, "Walk." And they walked.

--------------------- **INSIGHTS** ---------------------

- Enjoy all the celebrations. There will be birthdays, weddings and holidays—don't miss any of them because of Alzheimer's.

- Have faith in your loved one. Resist the natural temptation to pull back too far or set strict limits on celebrations or get-togethers. Mike repeatedly taught me that he could do more than I thought he could do . . . if I just gave him the chance.

- It's true that things are not always perfect for those who have Alzheimer's. I learned that it was okay to let go of perfect. Things don't have to be perfect to be meaningful.

- Sometimes the shortest words are all that's required. Kathleen knew not to confuse her dad with too much information. Her simple word "walk" could be a metaphor for the journey you take together with Alzheimer's. Just go ahead and "walk" with your loved one—and I promise you that good things will happen along the way.

CHAPTER 35

MIKE'S GIFT FOR THE BABY

*Now we move on to a sweet story
about Grandpa Mike wanting to buy
a special mystery gift for his future
grandchild.*

THE YEAR AFTER MIKE WALKED OUR DAUGHTER DOWN
THE aisle at her wedding, we heard the joyful news: Kathleen was
expecting a baby!

It was now seven-and-a-half years after Mike was diagnosed. He
was still walking, and we were still able to be out and about enjoying our days. And, of course, Mike was thrilled to hear about this
new baby entering our lives. But his ability to express his thoughts
was really starting to decline.

One morning a few months before the baby was due, he said,
"We have to get the baby something." I asked what he had in mind,
and all he said was, "You know. All babies need it."

Hmm, a mystery. I then asked him, "Mike, what does it look
like?" And he answered again, "You know, babies need it."

At that point I started going down the list. I asked him about baby
beds, baby clothes, baby toys. "No, no, no," none of those was right.

This back-and-forth guessing game went on for days, then weeks,
then months. By now, Mike and I were both thoroughly frustrated
and annoyed by our inability to identify the exact gift he wanted for
our grandchild.

In desperation, I finally said, "Let's go look in a baby store, maybe
you will see it there." I had high hopes that we could use the pointing technique, but I cautioned him, "Mike, if we don't see it at the

store, then we will just have to give up and find a different gift."

So off we went to Walmart, with two positive attitudes. We looked at virtually everything in the baby department that day, but none was right. "You know what babies need," Mike said for the hundredth time. Problem was I still didn't have a clue.

We left the store with Mike disappointed and me resigned that we would never figure this out, and it was time to stop talking about it. I worried that this was a new level of ongoing confusion, one that we would have to learn how to handle on a regular basis in the future.

HOW I FINALLY LEARNED WHAT BABIES NEED

A week or two went by with no more discussion about what babies need; Mike knew I was now officially done with that conversation. Then a Lamaze Getaway Retreat rolled around and it was time for me to leave for the weekend to teach it.

I made all the usual arrangements to have caring people with Mike while I was away. Stephanie would have the Sunday morning time slot. We decided our meeting place would be Starbucks near the shopping center at 9:00 a.m. Sunday morning. The handoff worked fine, I hugged Mike goodbye, and looked forward to seeing him later that day at the end of the retreat.

When I returned to pick Mike up at Starbucks I was surprised to see Stephanie's husband Chris sitting with Mike with a Walmart bag on their table. As Chris handed the bag to me he remarked, "Stephanie said this is something Mike wanted."

I looked in the bag and there was a package of brightly-colored children's alphabet blocks—you know the ones, the little square blocks with pictures on one side, letters and numbers on the other.

Mike did not act like this was something we had been attempting to purchase—forever. He just looked at me quite proudly. For he knew, as he had always known, that "this is what all babies need."

Needless to say, this required a phone call to Stephanie. She explained that Mike had told her he wanted something for the baby and they went to the same Walmart that Mike and I had gone to before. This time, however, Mike spotted the blocks and knew right away that this is what he had wanted all along.

Today, our grandchildren still love to play with the little wooden alphabet blocks from Grandpa Mike. Watching them play gives me such joy. They giggle and laugh, and I smile. It makes me think of the blocks that our children had when they were young. And reminds me of the bigger blocks that Mike handmade for our son Patrick when he got older. Blocks were a favorite toy for our children and now they are a favorite of our grandchildren.

Mike was right all along. He really *did* know what babies need.

----------------------------------- INSIGHTS -----------------------------------

- I'm glad that Mike did not give up on something he wanted, even at this advanced date in his illness. At this point in the journey, there was so little that he truly desired or requested. This gift for the baby had been important to him, and he had stuck with it.

- This was a reminder for me to continue hanging in there with my husband Mike. For when Mike won, it was such a big reward for both of us.

- I knew that Mike did not want to be difficult or create problems for me and yet sometimes it was hard to remember that. His persistence in searching for the blocks reminded me that I needed to always listen patiently and keep doing my part, especially when I was feeling frustrated with him.

- A reminder for you: don't forget that your circle of friends and family can help you solve the little problems and the big ones too—just as Stephanie and Chris had helped Mike and me with the baby gift.

- Mike often surprised me by how much he remembered and how much he knew. Believe in your partner, stay open for signs of deeper awareness, and your loved one will surprise you too.

CHAPTER 36

LITTLE RILEY AND GRANDPA MIKE HIT IT OFF RIGHT AWAY

*Some families might be reluctant
to have little children around
someone with Alzheimer's, but our
family felt just the opposite.*

HER NAME WAS RILEY ROSE and she immediately became a new and beautiful light in Mike's life. Our first grandchild came into the world in late January, the beginning of Mike's eighth year of illness. Because his abilities had significantly declined, I worried that Alzheimer's might prevent him from bonding with Riley. Instead, here's what happened:

The day Riley was born, Mike and I took the early morning ferry to the Ballard Swedish Hospital birthing center in Seattle. We were both excited to see our daughter Kathleen and to meet the new baby.

At the hospital, Mike and I waited patiently with our son Patrick, who had arrived with a big bouquet of flowers for his sister—and soon it was time for us to enter the birthing suite. I guided Mike to the chair by the bed, and our daughter immediately held out her arms with the most precious gift of all to her dad. With my arms cradled around his, Mike received our beautiful granddaughter while looking up at me to be sure he was doing it just right—and he was.

Tears of joy filled my eyes. It was one of those magic moments in life, and the beginning of a priceless relationship between little Riley and Grandpa Mike.

I understand why some families might be reluctant to have little children around someone with Alzheimer's, but our family felt just the opposite. In fact, when our daughter went back to work a few weeks after Riley's birth, Mike and I offered to babysit one day a week. It was a commitment we were able to continue every week for the last two-and-a-half years of Mike's life—and I'm so glad we did.

Having an exuberant toddler in our home during the final years of Mike's illness was an amazing experience. It was ironic to watch Riley's abilities increase as Mike's were decreasing, ever mindful of the gifts this precious new life brought to Mike and our family.

Over the next two-and-a-half years I watched Grandpa Mike and Riley learn to love each other, have empathy for each other, miss each other when they were separated, and most of all have fun together. Mike looked forward to their special day each week and so did Riley. She arrived with a smile, and when she learned to crawl she always went looking for Grandpa Mike if he was not near.

I have learned that laughter is not a cure for Alzheimer's but it is definitely a magical remedy or potion. The first year, Riley and Mike found their own ways of playing together, with Mike always smiling and Riley soon learning to smile back. Despite Alzheimer's, they learned their own renditions of Peek-a-boo, Little Piggy and Patty-cake, and enjoyed nursery rhymes and children's music together.

Oh sometimes there was crying, but Mike was never put off by Riley's tears, just concerned for this beautiful little girl who was simply doing all that babies do while he fell more in love with her every day. Along the way little Riley made us both laugh and giggle, and her baby hugs and kisses gave us joy for today and hope for tomorrow.

During the last months of Mike's life when his needs increased and his emotions could be unpredictable, I had Stephanie come and help me on the days Riley came to visit. In this way we were able to keep little Riley and Grandpa Mike at play.

I only remember two times when Mike had a meltdown and Riley had to be scurried into the next room for a bit. In both cases Riley did not seem to be upset by the situation. Later, when Riley and I sat on Grandpa's bed together, I explained to her that Grandpa Mike sometimes roars like a lion. Riley seemed to understand and think that was okay.

⇀ FROM MY JOURNAL ↼

RILEY AT 6 WEEKS OLD
(THE BEGINNING OF MIKE'S EIGHTH YEAR)

Mike is lovely with Riley. Big smiles for her and lovely little talks.
"You are so cute."
"You are so pretty."
"I'm your Papa."
He whistles for her and looks concerned when she cries.

RILEY AT 2 MONTHS

Riley is a wonderful part of our life. Mike held her at the end of her long nap today. He is so gentle and loving with her. Interesting how I am not writing about stress with Mike. I think it is because of my time with Riley, and the wonderful opportunity it gives me to connect with Kathleen.

RILEY AT 9 MONTHS

Mike really loves Riley and is so careful with her. When I went into the bathroom and Riley began to cry, Mike talked to her and all was fine. He often keeps her company in the living room, sitting on the bench, while I am watching from the kitchen.

~

Michael and Riley had great fun while sitting at the table. Riley would drop a spoon and Mike would pick it up and then have a great laugh together. After about 10 times, he would sometimes hide the spoon from Riley under his arm or make the spoon go in circles before she got it—all fun for both.

~

What a strange moment in time: Riley Rose at 9 months developing skills weekly while Michael is slowly losing his abilities.

Riley now crawls and pulls herself up very efficiently. She knows her name and can locate me from another room, crawling and looking around the corner for me.

Mike is very tuned into Riley and frequently wants to know "where is she?" Before we get up I often tell him what we are doing that day. When I say "Riley is coming," he is ready to get up quickly— right now!

RILEY AT 10 MONTHS

Riley tried to crawl out the back door. Grandpa held still while she crawled over his foot and yet bent down to try and hold her back while telling her "No"—so cute. They then sat on the bench in the carport together. After Riley left for the day, Mike laughed and said, "I's still looking for her."

RILEY AT 16 MONTHS

Riley is so patient with Grandpa. Pulled out his chair and patted it for him to sit. Walked like Grandpa and made me laugh. Puts Grandpa's hand in the sandbox. Takes toys to him and always looks for him when she arrives.

RILEY AT 18 MONTHS

Riley is so tuned into Mike and his emotions. When I returned from work, Mike was crying. Riley wanted me to stop everything and soothe her Grandpa.

RILEY AT 26 MONTHS

It was a lovely Easter with 14 dinner guests. Late in the afternoon Riley noticed Mike was sitting across the room all by himself; she came and took me by my hand to Grandpa. She patted his forearm and wanted me to interact with him. Her little hand on his big arm—so cute. I continue to think children and seniors go together.

(A room full of adults, but little Riley was the one looking out for Mike.)

RILEY AT 28 MONTHS OLD
(TWO WEEKS BEFORE MIKE DIED)

Riley still engages Grandpa. "Grandpa push." She wanted him to push the bird book to make bird sounds. She took her doll to show Grandpa and asked the doll to hold Grandpa's hand.
We spent the day in our room with Grandpa, played tent, looked out at boats and birds, and named people in Grandpa's photo album, all in all a lovely day. When it was time to go home, Riley gave Grandpa her doll.

WHAT CHILDREN TEACH US ABOUT ALZHEIMER'S

Alzheimer's is complicated but children teach us how to keep the main things the main things. Little children are amazing in their ability to love without preconditions or judgment. They have no preconceived ideas of what we should look like or be like, they simply accept our differences. They do not come into life with fear or suspicion, they come with a clean slate ready to meet the world and the people who love them, including those with Alzheimer's.

Some fear that children will not understand when we are ill or behave differently from others, and yet the children themselves seem to roll with the unexpected and accept life's surprises as they navigate the world they enter. They can even learn about Alzheimer's in this way, too, if we just give them the chance.

Riley's parents taught her how to be empathetic by being kind and loving to her. But Riley also learned about empathy by watching Nana Rosie (me) and other members of the family respect and honor Mike while he dealt courageously with Alzheimer's.

Even before she could run or talk, Riley understood how to relate positively to a grandpa with Alzheimer's who clearly loved her:

√ Riley knew that Grandpa walked slowly, so it was good to wait patiently for him. Later, when he needed a wheelchair, that was okay with her, too, because he was still Grandpa and we loved him.

√ She knew that sometimes you had to wait your turn when Grandpa needed help from Nana Rosie.

√ She knew that Grandpa couldn't always talk, but he could still smile and play his harmonica and sometimes whistle.

√ She learned it was fun to have tea parties with Grandpa and build tents in his room.

√ She understood that Grandpa would even play with her when he was ill. All a little girl had to do was hand him her doll and he would dutifully hold her.

I often think about the effect Grandpa Mike had on Riley. Does she still hold memories of kindness, joy, courage and love of someone dealing with Alzheimer's and of those caring for him? Will those memories translate into a lifetime of reaching out to others in difficulty? If so, I think that, too, is part of Mike's legacy.

Seven months after Mike died, another new grandbaby came into our lives. Riley's little brother was named Michael Langdon, but we all called him Gavin. Mike was no longer with us, and yet little Gavin would still get to know all about his Grandpa Mike through the memories and stories we often share. Today, Riley and Gavin continue to bring joy, laughter and hope to our home as the circle of life continues—and the memories of Grandpa Mike remain ever-present.

INSIGHTS

- I was afraid that Alzheimer's would prevent Mike and me from being active grandparents; I am forever thankful that Mike, Kathleen, Sam, Riley, and I did not let that happen.

- To whom it may concern: Please don't deny grandparents who have Alzheimer's the joy of their grandchild—be it a day, an hour, or just a few minutes at a time.

- "Savor the moment" was an important part of how Mike and I managed our journey with Alzheimer's. In the beginning we had no idea how long we would actually be able to babysit Riley, but by living in the moment we ended up having a glorious experience each week for the last two-and-a-half years of Mike's life.

- Mothers today are working outside their homes more than ever and often rely on grandparents to help with childcare. I hope this book makes the case that, if given a chance, Alzheimer's couples can still be of help in raising their grandchildren.

- Making memories starts early and lasts forever. At age five Riley told me that she could click her tongue, but could not whistle. She then went on to recall, Grandpa could whistle!

- At age six Riley noticed that I was enjoying a cup of tea with Mike's old 'no-handle' mug. "I like that cup," she said. I asked her why. She said, "Because it was Grandpa's."

- At age seven when Riley and I took deck chairs downstairs backwards, she said this is how you could take Grandpa down the stairs in his wheelchair. Exactly.

- Lesley Stahl of *60 Minutes'* fame writes in her book *Becoming Grandma* about her husband Aaron who has Parkinson's. One night, after Aaron had been tremoring and falling down, he propped their little granddaughter Jordan on his knees. "Giddyup!" he said, making her arms and legs dance. He laughed. She smiled back. It looked as though she was curing him. Mike, too, had a positive "reset" whenever he was around our granddaughter Riley.

- Martha and Mary is an innovative care facility not far from my home on Bainbridge Island. They provide memory care for senior citizens and also have a nearby pre-school and childcare center. For more than twenty years the caregivers at Martha and Mary have made arrangements for the children to visit the seniors often. Based on watching the wonderful relationship that Mike and Riley shared, I think this is a successful model that other care facilities and families should consider.

MIKE & ME

PART IX

~

Nourishing the Spirit

CHAPTER 37

KEEP THE MUSIC PLAYING

Music is therapy. It connects us in
ways that no other medium can.
It reaches in and touches our heart-
strings. It acts as medicine.
—Macklemore

THROUGHOUT MIKE'S ILLNESS I MADE SURE that his favorite songs and music were always near at hand, and for good reason. A growing body of research indicates that music can serve as an effective therapy for people with dementia, making a significant difference in their speech, motor skills, and overall mood.

It is said that music has the potential to soothe Alzheimer's patients, decreasing anxiety, tearfulness, and even combative behavior. I can personally vouch for that.

Many care facilities today have established an ongoing music program and some even have a music therapist who is trained to discover just the right music for each individual. For example, Mike's favorite music was classical, which his mother claimed was the result of her playing Bach, Mozart and other classical masters when he was a baby.

Mike also enjoyed more contemporary artists such as The Three Tenors and Anne Murray. So, throughout his years with Alzheimer's, I played classical music for him at home, and I also kept CDs of Anne Murray and the Tenors in the car to soothe and entertain us on the road.

WHEN WORDS FAIL

Two hundred years ago, Hans Christian Andersen, the beloved children's author, observed that, "When words fail, music continues to speak." Andersen could've been referring to Alzheimer's patients. It is simply remarkable to realize that some people who have Alzheimer's can continue to play beautiful music just as they did many years before, even though they are no longer able to speak or communicate in other ways.

A dramatic example is country music star Glen Campbell. The legendary voice of country hits such as "Rhinestone Cowboy" and "Wichita Lineman," Campbell was diagnosed with Alzheimer's in 2006. Incredibly, even as his ability to speak declined, Campbell's genius with music continued virtually full force. He was able to keep singing and playing for nearly six years after diagnosis. He even cut a new album and completed a one-year "farewell" concert tour with his adult children performing alongside him—even while his non-musical abilities were rapidly fading. He died in 2017, but his courage and spirit in the face of Alzheimer's is an inspiration to all.

How was it possible for Campbell to maintain much of his musical brilliance for so long? According to Professor Alicia Ann Clair, the Director of Music Education at the University of Kansas, "A person's ability to engage in music, particularly rhythm playing and singing, is unique. It remains intact late into the dementia process because playing familiar music does not require cognitive functioning for success."

THE GIFT OF MUSIC FOR MIKE'S 70TH

Years before Mike was diagnosed we had moved from Southern California to Washington. During the move we left behind our outdated turn-style record player and all our favorite records. Now, twenty years later, Mike had Alzheimer's and I wanted those familiar records back in our life. Mike's 70th birthday was coming up, and that seemed like just the time to give him the nostalgic gift of music.

Mike was quite surprised when he opened his present —a small old-fashioned record player—at our little family birthday celebration. Then the boxes of old records were brought up from the basement. Soon the familiar strains of Grofé's "The Grand Canyon Suite" and many other of Mike's favorites echoed through the house, not only that day but for all the years that followed.

Mike loved having the old records back in our life, and the little single-play record player was easy for him to operate. We often asked each other to dance on the living room rug to Ray Anthony's "Dancing Over the Waves" or Billy Vaughn's "Tenderly." We soon learned we had to give up the dip, which could lead to a tumble because of Alzheimer's—but the music and dancing remained.

Sing-along music came into our life, too, as we sang along with Mitch Miller's album with oldies like "You're the Cream in My Coffee" or "When the Red Red Robin Goes Bob Bob Bobbin' Along."

And, of course, there was also the lullaby music that I discovered was perfect to help Mike go to sleep. There was something about the slow lullaby rhythm that allowed him to settle down for a nap or for the night and so became a comforting presence and ritual in those difficult last months.

According to the Alzheimer's Association, "Music can be powerful. It provides a way to connect, even after verbal communication has become difficult ... Even in the late stages of Alzheimer's, a person may tap a beat or sing lyrics to a song from childhood."

--------------------------------- **INSIGHTS** ---------------------------------

- After Mike was diagnosed with Alzheimer's, we did what he said he wanted us to do—we got on with our lives. And we never gave up on doing all that we could to fight Alzheimer's every step of the way. That included daily reading together, exercise, qigong, diet, vitamins, chalk art and, yes, definitely Mike's favorite music.

- Mike had sung in a boy's choir as a child and had a nice voice, but he had no musical training on an instrument. Now that he had Alzheimer's, it did not seem like the right time to introduce an instrument, but I bought him a harmonica and it proved to be great fun for him.

- More recently I have heard beautiful music played and sung by an Alzheimer's choir group. It's inspiring; I wish Mike had had the opportunity to join a choir like that.
- The list of "Musical Tips for Alzheimer's Patients" on the next page appears in similar form on several caregiver websites. My sincere thanks to whomever originally created this list, as it has been very helpful to me and others in the Alzheimer's community.

MUSICAL TIPS FOR ALZHEIMER'S PATIENTS

Early Stage of Alzheimer's

- Go out dancing or dance in the house.
- Listen to music your loved one liked in the past—whether swing or Sinatra or salsa.
- Experiment with various types of concerts and venues, giving consideration to endurance and temperament.
- If your loved one played an instrument in the past, encourage him/her to try it again.
- Compile a musical history of favorite recordings, which can be used to help in reminiscence and memory recall.

Middle Stage of Alzheimer's

- Use song sheets or a karaoke player so your loved one can sing along with old-time favorites.
- Play music or sing as your loved one is walking to improve balance or gait.
- Use background music to enhance mood.
- Opt for relaxing music—a familiar, non-rhythmic song—to reduce sundowning or behavior problems at bedtime.

Late Stage of Alzheimer's

- Utilize the music collection of old favorites that you made earlier.
- Do sing-alongs to tunes sung in your loved-one's generation.
- Play soothing music to provide a sense of comfort.

CHAPTER 38

THE BEST MEDICINE OF ALL

Laughter in the face of reality is
probably the finest sound there is.
In fact a good time to laugh
is any time you can.
—Linda Ellerbee

IN HIS 1979 BEST SELLER "ANATOMY OF AN ILLNESS," Dr. Norman Cousins introduced the world to the healing power of "laughter therapy." After years of pain and discouragement from a life-threatening illness, Dr. Cousins described how he finally helped heal himself by watching cartoons, Laurel & Hardy movies, and old "I Love Lucy" reruns.

A growing body of research supports the theory that laughter is a natural medicine that can improve the quality of life for patients with chronic illnesses such as cancer, arthritis and, yes, Alzheimer's.

Among other things, laughter can relax the body and mind, boost the immune system, trigger the release of endorphins, inspire hope, diffuse anger, and promote love, optimism and the will to live—all very important for Alzheimer's patients. Laughter is a vital part of the human survival kit, wrote Cousins. Best of all it's free, fun and available in unlimited supplies.

As Mike's wife, best friend and caregiver, I learned firsthand how important it was for Mike and me to infuse our lives with daily doses of joy and laughter, especially in the later years of the disease. In my journal entries I even had a pet name for it—the "Perk Factor."

These lovely perks came to us from a variety of sources and were always a bright spot in the Alzheimer's experience. While I cannot say laughter cured Mike, I can say it made a huge difference in the quality of the journey. Here I share a few of those golden moments with you.

SOME FAVORITE PERK-UPS

It happened early in the ninth year of Mike's illness. At that point Mike was still walking and talking some, but the sadness of the disease could get us down. One night Mike was watching television in the next room. Suddenly I heard him laughing and then he called out to me, "You should come see this."

Soon I was at his side and we were both laughing out loud as Victor Borge—the zany piano virtuoso—ran through his hilarious comedy routine. It felt good for Mike and me to be laughing.

When the commercial came on to buy the Victor Borge CD, we got out the credit card and placed our order. Like Norman Cousins watching his Laurel & Hardy movies, Mike watched his favorite Victor Borge CD over and over the next year and a half. He especially enjoyed sharing it with guests or other caregivers. I remember one delightful volunteer with a very French accent. She and Mike would laugh out loud at that Borge CD together and even danced to the music with Mike in his wheelchair. It was so good for his spirits, and mine too.

There was also a noticeable "perk up" whenever our son Patrick would come from the city to visit. Patrick had a way of getting his dad to crack a smile. Mike would even perk up just by hearing that Pat was coming over for the day.

Kathleen, of course, added her own special perk each time she came by the house to give her dad a hug and drop off baby Riley for the day. These were sweet little visits and on those days we treasured the pure joy of a baby's laughter in our home.

HOW GOOD FRIENDS BRING HOPE AND LAUGHTER

Hats off to Marilyn and Claudia, our longtime friends from San Pedro, California. These two big-hearted women flew up to Seattle three times in the final months of Mike's life.

Talk about perk-ups! When these ladies came, there were always lots of hugs and kisses, stories of long ago, good-natured ribbing, hardy laughter and, of course, good smells from the kitchen. They made our home come alive with love, laughter and good food, which was just what we needed at this late stage of the disease.

The last months had become more difficult physically and emotionally for Mike, and his frustration often led to emotional meltdowns. It wasn't until after Marilyn and Claudia's third and final visit in April, just six weeks before Mike would no longer be with us, that I realized something extraordinary happened whenever the ladies were here: namely, Mike would never have a meltdown.

Then and now I wonder why. Was it because Mike could hold it together with company when he had to? Or was it because his brain was getting the much-needed endorphins from the laughter, friendship, and moments of joy that made it easier for him to cope?

Looking back, I do know that Mike and I were both more hopeful and joyful whenever friends, family, or caregivers arrived with love in their hearts and made us laugh.

CHASING DEPRESSION AWAY

In April of Mike's last year, while Marilyn and Claudia were here, we invited our mutual friends Dave and Kathy to come to our home. We had a lovely time together with lots of storytelling and laughter about old times. We went to the Japanese memorial, stopped to feed the ducks, and returned home in time for Mike to have his all-important afternoon nap. Then we all enjoyed a family-style meal together!

The menu that day was thoughtfully designed especially for Mike, including his favorite meatloaf, soft roasted vegetables, fresh Blackbird Bakery bread, and yummy home-made apple pies, all served with a hearty red wine. I was a little hesitant about more wine for Mike, so when Claudia offered more I declined for him.

But Mike raised his head, opened his eyes wide, and lifted his right arm. Claudia looked at me and said, "I think Mike wants more wine" and he had it! We had a wonderful night with friends, a great deal of laughter, and a little too much wine.

That was a long, busy day for Mike, but there was no meltdown as I feared might happen; we just had fun, forgot about Alzheimer's for the moment, and let the laughter and positive feelings flow.

As I write about the perk factor, I can't help but wonder about the reasons behind the depression that often comes with Alzheimer's.

We know that when parents become depressed, their baby can also become depressed. Knowing the effect that a parent's emotional state can have on a baby naturally makes me wonder about the relationship between the caregiver and the Alzheimer's patient. Is it possible that if we as caregivers become depressed, then we may inadvertently play a role in making the one we love depressed?

To put it more positively, if we as caregivers are happy, can that make a difference in the daily happiness of those we are caring for? Perhaps there are studies out there that can help answer these questions. I can only tell you that, thanks in large part to our dear friends and family, Mike and I experienced many golden moments of love and laughter in our home, and it made all the difference for us.

⤳ FROM MY JOURNAL ⤶
FEBRUARY (YEAR 10)

Marilyn and Claudia were here for four days. It was a lovely visit and so very helpful. Special memories: Mike's greeting; he knew them and was glad they were here to see him. "I'm glad you come"... wonderful breakfasts together in our bedroom ... laughter and tears... sharing stories of past and present... he really enjoyed all the kisses and attention.

INSIGHTS

- The Alzheimer's Association reminds us that depression is very common among people with Alzheimer's, especially during the early and middle stages. Could it be that a little daily laughter therapy, especially with friends and family, might be an antidote?

- Some cancer treatment centers have introduced daily "laughter sessions" for their patients. After a laughter session patients have said things like, "I didn't even think about cancer while I was laughing, and that felt great!" Perhaps that can work for Alzheimer's couples too.

- With the high cost of prescription drugs these days, we can all benefit from a "natural therapy" like laughter, which is free.

- An article in *The New York Times* featured a group called "Nurses for Laughter" at Oregon Health Sciences University. The nurses all wear buttons that say: "Warning: Humor May Be Hazardous to Your Illness." I think that's a good affirmation and reminder for Alzheimer's couples too.

CHAPTER 39

KISSES AND HUGS CONTINUE

*Maintaining little rituals of love
and friendship means a lot when you
and your loved one are living
with Alzheimer's.*

DEALING WITH ALZHEIMER'S AT HOME can be unpredictable and even chaotic at times. In a sometimes hectic environment, it's comforting to have little rituals and routines that you and your loved one can count on and look forward to.

For example, in the years before Alzheimer's, Mike and I would always share a goodbye kiss on the days I went to work and a hello kiss when I came back in the evening. It was so thoughtful the way Mike made a point of giving me a warm welcome whenever I returned from work. He would usually step away from the TV, greet me at the door and ask me about my day. And of course there was always that warm hug and a kiss.

As Alzheimer's progressed, our departures and reunions had even greater meaning. Our familiar little ritual helped reassure Mike that I would be gone for a time, but that I loved him and would soon return. Giving Mike that all-important goodbye kiss helped him stay connected to me and his world while I was gone.

Oh, sometimes, especially in the final year, there were tears, similar to what can happen when children don't want their parent to leave. That was sad for me, but I never avoided Mike's tears—or our good bye kiss—by simply slipping away or hoping he would not notice I was gone.

As Alzheimer's progressed, our circumstances changed but our familiar ritual remained intact. Even in the final months Sabina (our wonderful late- stage caregiver) made a point to have Mike ready to greet me in his wheelchair at the back door when I came home. Looking back I can remember driving home from the ferry at night, anticipating his cheerful greeting.

Remembering Mike's big smile and outstretched arms awaiting me still brings a smile to my face and tears to my eyes. Thanks to our continuing ritual, there were always hugs and kisses both day and night for Mike and me even in the very last days of our journey with Alzheimer's.

So don't forget your hugs and kisses whenever you depart or return. Make it a delightful tradition for you and the one you love— one that provides an important way to stay connected and keep a little daily romance and affection in your relationship.

───────────── **INSIGHTS** ─────────────

- In my research-based workshops for new parents and couples, I teach that kissing your loved one goodbye and hello is a ritual that enhances relationships.

- Teaching new parents the value of this simple ritual served as a constant reminder to me not to forget the importance for Mike and me.

- Be open to creating other rituals in your relationship, be it morning walks, afternoon tea or coffee times, or simply looking at the moon together each night—all of which are food for the spirit.

CHAPTER 40

ON FAITH AND PRAYER

*The feeling remains that God is
on the journey too.*
—St. Teresa of Avila

FAITH IS SUCH A PERSONAL THING. What I believe or don't believe is possibly quite different from what you believe or don't believe. And so I never presume to offer anyone spiritual advice. But I can say with certainty that Mike and I found renewed strength and comfort for our fight with Alzheimer's by turning to our church and our faith in new ways. It did not happen overnight, it happened over time, but I hope our experience will be helpful to you and your loved one now.

By the time Mike was told that he had Alzheimer's, we were long-time members of St. Barnabas Episcopal Church. St. B's (as it is affectionately called) was built in 1946 and sits atop a tree-lined hill on Bainbridge Island. It's a delightful example of an early Norman English brick church, with a square bell tower, beautiful stained-glass windows, and a peaceful outside memorial garden where the ashes of those who have passed are interred. If it sounds idyllic, I assure you it is all of that.

After retirement, Mike volunteered to help look after the memorial garden and was a good caregiver for those who had departed. He opened the little niches one by one, placing flowers on the ones that were in need. And he told me that he often had a little chat with those at rest as he tidied up the grounds.

Long before Alzheimer's entered our life, St. B's gave Mike and me a quiet and holy place to worship... a spiritual leader who was always there for us…a community of good-hearted people with similar values … and a place for friendship, laughter and community involvement.

As you might imagine, after Mike was diagnosed, we turned to our faith and our church in even deeper ways. It's no surprise that Alzheimer's made us more conscious of our mortality, and put us in closer touch with life and death. Here is where we drew the strength and courage we needed for the latter part of the journey.

THE GIFT OF PRAYER

Over our forty plus years of marriage, Mike and I had rarely prayed together. Prayer was something we did in church or at special family meals during the holidays, but not together at home.

About a year before Mike died, however, I began to kneel beside the bed at night and say prayers with him. I only wish we had started this daily prayer practice much earlier, for it soon became such an important part of our day.

Because I was out of practice, I started with the familiar Lord's Prayer, but soon found myself praying more easily and naturally. Novelist Anne Lamott once said there are only two kinds of prayer: "help me, help me, help me," and "thank you, thank you, thank you." Mike and I did both.

Every night I thanked God for all that we had, and I asked God for the privilege to continue caring for Mike in our home. Each day Mike and I also said prayers for those who had passed, for those who were suffering, and for all the men and women in our military.

At first I wasn't sure if Mike was fully present or aware of our prayers. Then one night, as I started to rise from my knees, I was surprised to hear him urgently call out, "The boys, the boys!" Hmm, I had clearly forgotten to pray for someone, but who? Then it came to me. "Are you talking about the men and women in the military?" I asked. His eyes widened and I happily told him he was right. Then I knelt again to properly finish our prayers.

Kneeling at our bed, holding Mike's hand, speaking softly, remembering those who were suffering more than ourselves, and being thankful for what we had (rather than what we had lost) was such a powerful way to end each day, especially during the final year.

NO NEED TO WAIT

In her beautiful book for cancer patients, author Vickie Girard reminds us: "Never forget that you have a toll-free, never-busy, direct line from your heart to God's ear." In other words, we don't need to wait for Sunday services or for evening prayers to have a word with God, we can call on Him anytime and anyplace, knowing that He hears us.

One day, during Mike's last months, my sister Gerri gave me a live example of this principle in action. That day a social worker and home healthcare nurse had made a visit to our home and were asking Mike questions which he was struggling mightily to answer. After a time he became upset and tearful, at which point Gerri calmly intervened with, "Can I say a prayer?" As we all held hands and my sister prayed softly, the tension in the room and for Mike subsided and the situation returned to normal. Again, this was a beautiful reminder that prayer is there for us anytime and anyplace—no waiting necessary.

A few nights later I needed that beautiful reminder. It happened in the morning around 2:00 AM. I had rolled back into my single bed after cuddling next to Mike in his hospital bed and woke with him thrashing his arms and crying out in a complete meltdown. I felt an adrenaline rush and responded quickly by switching on the lights and elevating the head of his bed.

With his arms continuing to flail, there was no way I could safely approach him, so I waited until I could tuck a little Lorazepam under his tongue. I then had to wait and just hope that his panic would pass. As I sat there, tense and distraught, I thought of Gerri and her easy way of praying. On the bookshelf next to me were some scriptures from St. B's services. I began to read them softly to Mike and was relieved to see how quickly he began to calm.

There in our little room at that moment I felt the presence of more than just us as the words flowed from the scriptures and we calmed together. As St. Teresa of Avila reminds us, "The feeling remains that God is on the journey too."

—————————————— **INSIGHTS** ——————————————

- Father Dennis at St. B's said that prayer clarifies what really worries us, what it is that we truly fear, and what it is that we honestly desire. And, in naming those, we come up with an orderly list of what really matters. And that seemed to be true for Mike and me.

- How Mike and I practiced our faith outwardly changed over our many years of marriage, but in the end we turned more and more to our faith for the strength to carry us through those last few months — and we were not denied.

PART X

~

Counting Our Blessings
in Year 9

CHAPTER 41

12 UNEXPECTED BLESSINGS
AT THIS LATE STAGE

*In the last full year of Mike's life, we
were still living together at home and
still enjoying most days in ways that
often defied conventional wisdom.*

WHEN MIKE WAS FIRST DIAGNOSED WITH ALZHEIMER'S we
were told that most people live just nine years after diagnosis. We
were also told that the last two years are typically spent in a 24-hour
care facility—but that was not our experience at all.

In year nine Mike was not only still alive, he was still living with
me at home, and we were still enjoying most days in ways that often
defied conventional wisdom and surpassed everyone's expectations.

Again, even in year nine, Mike was still Mike. Despite his severe-
ly diminished capacity, we could still connect with each other as
best friends and life partners. There was no question in my mind
that he still knew and loved me...that he still knew and loved his
family and close friends...that he still enjoyed and appreciated life's
simple pleasures...that he still understood and celebrated special
occasions...and he could still look forward to what the next day
would bring.

Here in this chapter I've outlined 12 ways that Mike defied the
usual Alzheimer's statistics and surpassed typical expectations in
the last full year of his illness. Some will be new stories and some
you will recall from past chapters, but each tells us how present
Mike was in this ninth year. This should be hopeful news for all Alzheimer's couples.

More than ever I am convinced that the home care regimen that Mike and I used resulted in many of the positive results we experienced throughout our journey with Alzheimer's. Equally important, I'm confident now that these same strategies and outcomes can be replicated in whole or in part by many other Alzheimer's couples.

12 POSITIVE OUTCOMES IN MIKE'S LAST FULL YEAR

1. In Mike's ninth year we were still able to travel.

Each year of Mike's illness I wondered if we could still make the drive to our beloved cabin in Montana, and each year I was pleasantly surprised when it happened. But making two trips in Mike's ninth year far exceeded anything I ever imagined. I am so grateful to family and friends who made those final trips possible by traveling with us and helping with Mike's care when it was needed.

2. In Mike's ninth year we continued to enjoy holidays and family celebrations.

For Mike's 75th birthday in May we had a party for him with 23 guests. Later that summer, much to my surprise, Mike told Patrick that he wanted another party. This time we invited friends from work and others he had not seen for a while. It was a brunch with finger foods to make it easy for Mike.

Some will ask, "What is the point of throwing a party if the person with Alzheimer's will not even remember the event?" My answer: Do we really care if our loved one remembers? Isn't it more important that he or she enjoys the moment and shares it with family and friends?

3. In Mike's ninth year we were still able to socialize.

Early in the ninth year I wondered if Mike would still want to go places and see people, but he assured me in his own way that he was still up for a little adventure and socializing. Among other things, we went to church, saw friends, and enjoyed lots of little outings together.

New Year's Day—the beginning of his last full year—we drove to Port Ludlow, had a picnic in the car, took a little walk, and ended with an Irish coffee in the inn, which was such a treat. I remember Mike laughing at funny little things, and telling me that I was beautiful, and that he loved me. It was a lovely day.

In the summer, my sister Patty and her family spent a month sailing Puget Sound and used our house as their home base. It was a busy month with lots of family, but one filled with love and laughter for Mike and me. We had such fun!

In the fall, Patty returned with her son Andy to help care for Mike while I taught a Getaway Weekend class. The three of them went to the Tacoma Art Museum, enjoyed meals out, and had an amazing weekend—all in the ninth year of Mike's illness.

4. In Mike's ninth year he still had really good days.
One Sunday, when I picked Mike up from his friend Stan's, he walked confidently out of the house and talked all the way home. We laughed together about whatever he was talking about. I couldn't figure out everything he was telling me, but I knew he had enjoyed a very good time. Coming so late in the disease, these surprising good days continued to happen here and there in year nine and caught me off guard.

5. In Mike's ninth year he still laughed and could make me laugh!
That we could still have fun and laugh this late in Mike's illness was such a pleasant surprise. Mike gets the credit here because early in the disease he made a conscious decision to look at the funny side of most situations rather then get upset—and he stuck with it.

Thanks to Mike we had the gift of laughter in our home all through the Alzheimer's journey. Even on Mike's seventy-fifth birthday he played the harmonica at a family get-together and made Donald Duck sounds, getting everyone to laugh.

In the summer of his ninth year, while at Quinn's Hot Springs in Montana, I gave Mike lots of instructions about what to do as we tried to get him out of the pool. He had everyone laughing when he replied, "Yes, Master."

On another day Mike heard me talking to a potential new caregiver on the phone. When I got off the phone, he informed me that when she came he was going to... and then he played limp in the wheelchair and acted like he was completely out of it. Oh my, he could make me laugh.

As I mentioned earlier, research tells us that those who learn to laugh at life's ups and downs typically live longer happier lives. Mike gives proof of that. Well into his final full year, he continued to defy Alzheimer's by laughing at the joyful things that happened in our home, especially when our granddaughter was with us.

6. In Mike's ninth year he remembered far more than I expected.
I was surprised whenever Mike remembered something that had happened recently. At this late stage of Alzheimer's I thought he might remember some past events but I was pleasantly surprised when he remembered more recent things.

One day, for example, I told Mike about a troubling incident at work. Later that night—out of the blue—he inquired about the outcome of the event at bedtime. His words were limited, but he was able to say, "Your work?" I figured out what he wanted to know and assured him, "It worked out fine." It was such a thoughtful question. Despite all that he was coping with himself, he just wanted to be sure everything was okay for me at work.

Mike awoke early one December morning in that ninth year. As we lay in bed together, I retold him the familiar love story of how we first met. At the end, I began to cry and then Mike, too, began to cry. I put my arms around him and we had our little cry together. Then I said, "I don't know why we are crying about our love story." Mike looked at me and said, "It is true." I did not expect Mike to remember our love story at that late stage; it was such a welcome surprise to discover that he did.

7. In Mike's ninth year he continued to care about our grand-daughter Riley and others.

My journal entries recount the many times Mike continued to show that his personal connection to the people he loved was still intact in year nine. Here are a few examples:

One day, when I was calling my sister, Mike spoke up and told me to tell her that he loved her.

Another day when Mike was on an outing with Stephanie he became sad and asked about baby Riley and wanted to go home. He knew Riley was coming that day and wanted to see her.

Yet another time as we talked in the kitchen Mike began to cry and said, "the girl." I asked if he was talking about Riley and he nodded. He was obviously concerned about her and I think it was connected to his awareness that he was dying. When I assured him that Riley's mom and dad take good care of her, he calmed.

8. In Mike's ninth year were still best friends and life partners.

In that final full year of his life Mike was still there for me to snuggle and talk to. I was not just his caregiver, I was still his wife and friend. I was selective about what I talked about because it could be confusing for him. But I could always tell him about my day and talk with him about what I knew had happened in his day too. Late in the year I knew he understood only portions of what I said, and yet I was still talking to him and he was still actively listening and trying to understand. My advice to all Alzheimer's couples: *Don't stop talking about life with one another just because the clarity of your conversation has changed.*

9. In Mike's ninth year he still showed empathy for others.

Empathy—the ability to understand and share the feelings of another—is one of humanity's most advanced and endearing qualities and something that not everyone exhibits. To see that Mike continued to care about the feelings of others at this late stage, and was concerned if others were in pain, was remarkable and beautiful.

Mike, of course, was especially concerned when little Riley cried, but his concern didn't stop there. When I was sick, Mike wanted to get help for me and said "she." I knew he meant our daughter Kathleen and told him that she was gone. He then said "Pat" a number of times and I knew he was still determined to find help for me.

Another time I remember stubbing my toe on the wheelchair and Mike reached for my hand looking very sad. He felt my pain!

10. In Mike's ninth year he still missed me when I was gone.
One day after his massage, Mike became agitated when he discovered I was gone. As always, I had told him earlier that I was leaving, but on this day he did not remember.

So the next time the massage therapist came I sat next to Mike during the massage. He frequently looked up to see that I was still nearby. At one point his left hand reached for mine—it was so touching. Mike asked for little, he just wanted to stay connected.

11. In Mike's ninth year he was not chronically grumpy or angry.
In the very first year of the disease, whenever Mike caught himself being grumpy, he typically said, "No, I am not going to be like that." Years later he would still shake his head and remind himself, "I am not going to do that." It was a choice, a commitment—and he stuck by his commitment to the end. This gives us hope that people with Alzheimer's can maintain some control over their emotions and choose their own attitude, even late in the illness.

12. In Mike's ninth year he still knew and loved his wife.
How could that be possible? With Alzheimer's, aren't you eventually supposed to lose awareness of the one you love? Be assured that it's not always that way. As you can see from my previous journal notes, Mike continued to demonstrate that he loved his wife and family throughout his illness. Here are just a few small but meaningful examples from his last full year of life that show we were still very much in love:

√ After I tucked Mike in bed one night and started to leave the room he said, "Honey." I returned and knelt beside the bed and he looked at me and said, "I love you."

√ One day, while I was in the city, I called home and asked to talk to Mike. I said, "I love you," and he clearly replied "I love you." What is so memorable about the simple words "I love you" from Mike is that they were so clear and sincere, not said in haste or without meaning.

√ Another way Mike showed his love was by expressing concern for my safety. Even in his ninth year, when I was not there, he feared that something might have happened to me. One day when I returned from work we had a little talk as we sat on the living room bench. He was tearful. In his own way he told me, "I thought you were gone, I didn't know what happened to you."

Mike continued to respond to my voice, touch, and presence throughout his ninth year. At that point my greatest wish was that it might be possible for our love and mutual awareness to continue even to the final day. Without question, Mike's love for me and his family—and our continuing love for each other—helped make this cruel disease more bearable.

INSIGHTS

- The biggest insight in the ninth year is that Mike was still Mike. He was still present with us—something I did not think would be possible in late Alzheimer's. As long as we reached out to him, and continued to believe he was still with us, he could respond and reach out to us too.

- It is easy to overlook that someone is still present when they cannot interact in the way we are used to. Instead, watch closely for any signs of awareness and you, too, will be surprised and rewarded with the resulting response and connection.

- Do not disregard or discount the little signs that your loved one is still engaged and in love with you—write them down so you can remember them in years to come. I am so glad now that I kept a journal throughout our Alzheimer's journey.

- Stay open, even to the very end, to the positive things that might happen (rather than worry about the negative things that you've been told will probably happen). Expect good things to happen and they very often will.

- Last but not least, focus every day on what your loved one can still do, rather than fret about what he or she can no longer do.

CHAPTER 42

A FAREWELL VISIT TO MOUNTAIN BROOK

*Traveling to our beloved Montana
cabin at this late stage seemed like an
impossible dream for Mike and me,
but two good friends showed up to
make the dream come true.*

THROUGHOUT THESE PAGES you have read how grateful we are for the good friends who accompanied Mike and me in both spirit and deed on this difficult journey. Truthfully, there is not room enough in this book to list all the thoughtful and creative ways in which people reached out to make a difference along the way—and usually without ever being asked.

To show you what I mean I have chosen one beautiful story for this chapter. I think this particular story—told by our good friend Margaret Gaines in her own words—speaks volumes. It shows what I mean when I say that it's the circle of friends and family who make it possible for couples like Mike and me to stand up to Alzheimer's— and to continue fulfilling our dreams and our lives. Margaret's story took place in the ninth year of Mike's illness. Here she recounts a heartwarming trip the four of us made to Montana—a trip that Mike and I would never have attempted alone at that late stage.

A FAREWELL VISIT TO MOUNTAIN BROOK
BY MARGARET GAINES

As time went on it became too difficult for Rosalys to take Mike to their cabin in Montana alone. So, my husband Mike and I decided to fly up to Seattle and then drive to Montana—the four of us!

When we arrived at Mountain Brook, we all entered the family cabin that Mike's dad had built, pushing Mike's wheelchair up the ramp that Rosalys had thoughtfully installed.

Here we were, four old friends together again, but now one of us was coping with all the symptoms of advanced Alzheimer's. And yet, sitting in that cabin together, I saw in Mike's face a distinct smile, a knowing recollection of previous happy times! We stayed a few days, immersed in the warmth of our friendship and the quiet beauty of our natural surroundings.

At one point, Rosalys and I broke away to go down to the woodshed for a good cry. There my friend expressed her greatest hope—that she could continue to care for Mike at home until the very end, just as they had planned nine years before.

We returned to the cabin to find our two Mikes sitting out on the deck with the brook gurgling beneath them. My Mike is an artist and I noticed he had placed a block of wood and a pencil on the table. I watched as he drew his friend just sitting there enjoying the sounds of Mountain Brook. Today, Mike's image on that block of wood is still displayed in a special corner of the cabin. It's a wonderful memory of Mike's last trip with his old friends to the beloved cabin his dad built.

At the end of our stay, I wrote this entry in the cabin guest book: "Thank you Mike and Rosalys for a friendship that flowed like a mountain brook over hard spots and smooth places, but mostly deep in our hearts. Oh what a privilege my dear friends!"

Love, Margaret

WHY I FINALLY HIRED A PROFESSIONAL CAREGIVER

*In August of Mike's last year,
I wrote in my journal: "Sabina has
entered our lives as a caregiver.
How lucky we are."*

IT WASN'T UNTIL MIDWAY THROUGH YEAR NINE of Mike's illness that I finally decided to bring in a professional caregiver. You might ask why I waited so long. The simple answer is that Mike did not want to bring another person into our home. I honored his wishes as long as I could, but I almost waited too long. I hope you will benefit from what we learned. Here's what happened:

The summer of Mike's last year was a real crunch time for me and our circle of support. A whole series of events conspired all at once to make things more difficult. Mike was losing his ability to walk, Patrick was moving away to the East Coast for work, and Kathleen had alerted me it was now too difficult to care for dad by herself.

Throughout Mike's illness I had tried my best to look ahead—to constantly anticipate what might happen next and be ready for it. But in this case I had allowed our situation to get close to a crisis. I simply did not see that everything was on the verge of becoming too much for me until it was happening. If we were going to keep things together, I had to find and hire professional help immediately.

HOW WE FOUND THE RIGHT CAREGIVER

There are basically two options for hiring a professional caregiver. You can go through an agency, or you can find and hire a caregiver yourself. In our case, I asked Karen (who ran the support group I attended) for advice. She provided a list of experienced professional caregivers—and I took it from there.

Keep in mind that there are two things to look for in a caregiver: one is competency, and the other is chemistry. You need both. The first two caregivers we tried had good references (competency), but neither worked out for us on a personal level (chemistry.) One was not a good fit for Mike and the other was not a good fit for me. But I didn't give up. On our third try Sabina entered our lives and we couldn't have found a better fit.

Sabina was from Germany, tallish, about my height and ten years my junior. She had multiple degrees including a nursing degree, had worked as a nurse's aide in the U.S., had experience in long-term care facilities, and had now decided to specialize in home care. She was oh-so-capable and, equally important, she, Mike and I clicked right away.

Sabina had multiple clients so we had to agree on the days and hours that she could work for us. Because I taught classes on Tuesdays, that was the day we would start with. If all went well, she would also help on the weekends when I taught my Getaway classes.

As always, cost was a factor for Mike and me, but Sabina was not really open to negotiating her fee. She knew her value and we sensed it too. As we quickly learned, she was worth every penny.

On August 25th of Mike's last year, I wrote in my journal: *"Sabina has entered our lives as a caregiver for Mike. How lucky we are. Last night was her first night with Mike while I went to teach. She not only cared for Mike, but did laundry and vacuumed. I felt completely at ease leaving Mike with her."*

THE BEST CAREGIVERS LISTEN AND TEACH

While I originally thought we were mainly hiring Sabina to help with Mike's physical care, it turned out that she did much more than that. She was the type of person who would listen when things were difficult, offer moral and emotional support, and give me praise and encouragement when I needed it most.

I was more than willing to do all that Mike required, but I had no experience in caring for someone with Alzheimer's at the end of life. What's the easiest and safest way for a woman to move a man from a wheelchair to a chair? How do you manage a shower or get someone out of bed when they can no longer stand? What would the end of life be like for Mike?

Sabina had seen all this and more, and could show me how to do things safely and efficiently. Yes, she was both a great listener and a caring teacher—and that's just what I needed at this critical time in our Alzheimer's journey.

It helped, too, that she alerted me about what we might expect around the next bend. Knowing what might happen was helpful for me; it eliminated some of my fears and helped Mike and me make the most of our final months together.

A CHANGE FOR THE BETTER

When a professional caregiver like Sabina enters your circle, there will be changes in your home, yes—but it's all okay. Blankets may be folded differently, food and dishes may be stored in different places, windows may be opened or closed, and of course your loved one will now have a new friend. But, again, you will no doubt discover that it is all okay.

Now that Sabina was onboard, I noticed that I was breathing a little deeper, sleeping a little better, and was pretty sure that I could continue my work, and I was glad of that.

Mike continued to prefer that I be with him, but he also understood that sometimes I needed to be away from home. So he and Sabina learned to enjoy their days together and to manage just fine when I couldn't be there.

Even though Mike was becoming quieter and less communicative, Sabina and I were careful to honor his presence and to include him as fully as possible in our conversations. Instead of talking "about" Mike, either in person or behind his back, we made a constant effort to talk openly "with" him and "to" him, even at this late stage in his illness.

There were times when I personally turned to Sabina for emotional encouragement. That usually happened privately by the kitchen door just as she was ready to depart. With Sabina, I knew it was always okay for me to cry, feel sad, or wonder out loud if I could do all that was necessary for Mike. But I didn't want to do too much of that in front of him, for he was already working hard at his part, doing the best he could with a difficult situation. My role was to support and love him and not get caught up in how hard it was getting for him or for me. Sabina allowed me to cry in a safe space.

That I never saw Sabina speak unkindly to Mike was a big deal for me. Drawing from the Gottman "Couples' Relationship" workshop I teach, I knew that certain ways of speaking to your partner are destructive to the relationship. These include criticism, defensiveness, contempt or stonewalling. I did not do these things with Mike, either before or during our Alzheimer's journey, and I expected the same from Sabina and others who provided care for him.

I am happy to report there was never an interaction between Mike and Sabina that I felt could have been handled better; she was now in our circle and we were so glad she was.

INSIGHTS

- Having a professional caregiver can be compared to couples having a birth doula. What sets the doula apart from what other loved ones can provide is that she has done this before and knows what lies ahead.

- It can be difficult to find the right caregiver on your own. I was lucky that my support group had a list. There are, however, excellent private companies that can connect you.

- When looking for a caregiver, find one that can commit to the hours you need...has good chemistry with both you and your loved one...and will give you both the support and encouragement you need.

- Not all caregivers are right for everyone. Keep looking until you find the right fit. Don't hesitate to make a change.

- Don't wait too long to bring in a professional caregiver. In our case, it would have been better if Mike and I had acted sooner.

CHAPTER 44

SAVING MIKE FROM BECOMING BEDRIDDEN

As more and more couples make the decision to manage Alzheimer's at home, we are learning what to do when our loved ones can no longer get out of bed on their own.

I MENTIONED THIS TIP IN CHAPTER 23, but it's worth providing more details here to help you with this important topic. There comes a time when a person with Alzheimer's can no longer get out of bed or stand safely on their own. Sadly, many spend the remainder of their last year or more of life stranded in bed. I was determined not to have that happen to Mike, but how could I get him safely in and out of bed by myself at home?

Blessed Sabina, our caregiver, had the answer: "You need a Sit-to-Stand machine." I had never heard of such a thing, but I called hospice and then the medical supply store and soon we had a Sit-to-Stand machine on order for our home.

You can see photos and videos of this brilliant little battery-powered "lift" online. There are various models, but here's a basic description of the one Mike and I used:

Picture two tall metal "Ls" about two-and-a-half feet apart with a flat platform connecting them at the bottom. The L-shaped metal base is rolled under the bed (you need a hospital bed for this). The top of the "L" has two handlebars for the person to hold on to. There is a harness that goes around the person and hooks to the handlebars. With a push of the button the battery powered winch causes the handlebars and harness to rise, pulling the person right off the bed and up to their feet.

Mike's job was to simply hang on to the handlebars and stand up properly when the winch rose, which he was proud to do and worthy of all the praise that I always gave. Once Mike was up on his feet, the machine could be wheeled out from under the bed and I could use it to roll him safely and easily to any room in the house.

WHAT A DIFFERENCE IT MADE

The machine was truly magical. For months I had struggled getting Mike out of bed or out of his wheelchair, and now suddenly I could do it easily by myself. Once Mike was on his feet I could lower him into his wheelchair or roll him easily around the house.

The best part about the lift was seeing how happy it made Mike to be tall and upright again. Thanks to the Sit-to-Stand machine, he was no longer stuck in a wheelchair or a bed. Not only did he look like the old Mike standing tall, but he could breathe better, his muscles could stretch, his internal organs could settle where they belonged, and his feet could feel his weight again.

Mike and I both liked the Sit-to-Stand as did Riley. At age two, she loved seeing her grandpa standing again and looked forward to her occasional turn on the magic machine when Grandpa was not having his. We now had new laughter rolling around our house.

FIGHTING THE TEMPTATION TO STAY IN BED

As more and more couples make the decision to manage Alzheimer's at home, I think the Sit-to-Stand machine will become a more familiar and beloved piece of equipment.

Currently far too many people become bedridden simply because their caregivers are unable to get them in and out of bed throughout the day. A simple mechanical aid like the Sit-to-Stand changes all that.

Because of the Sit-to-Stand machine, I think Mike stayed engaged with the world for a much longer time. Thanks to the machine, it was possible to transfer Mike to his wheelchair, which allowed him to still go outside on the deck, still take car rides, and still enjoy meals at the dining room table when the family was present.

Because of the machine, Mike no longer laid in bed all day. His body was stronger and more upright than before. And he was able to avoid painful bedsores and infection.

Finally, the Sit-to-Stand machine made everyday care safer and easier for the caregiver (me or Sabina). My only regret is that we did not know about it sooner. Before we ordered the Sit-to-Stand, Mike had a few falls while I was attempting to move him; in those cases, we were both at risk of injury.

Quite frankly, without the Sit-to-Stand, Mike would have had to spend his last months in bed, which would have made both of us prisoners to this illness. Instead, our life continued on with simple pleasures: getting out of bed to greet the day, looking at the clouds, seeing children at play, hearing the birds, enjoying the sunshine, and being with people we loved.

─────────── **INSIGHTS** ───────────

- I am happy to report Mike never had a bedsore of any kind.

- Thanks in large part to the Sit-to-Stand machine, Mike was up and out of bed each and every day until the last week of his life.

- You can learn more about Sit-to-Stand machines online but be sure to ask your physician or care provider which stand will work best for your needs.

CHAPTER 45

CELEBRATING OUR 45TH WEDDING ANNIVERSARY

*I knew that Year 10 would mark our
last anniversary and I wanted
to make it special.*

THROUGH THE YEARS, MAY 21 had always been our special day—the day Mike and I had been married at All Saints Episcopal Church more than four decades before.

But when March and April of Mike's tenth and final year of Alzheimer's rolled around, it did not seem he would even be with us in May. Still, I watched with anticipation, hoping we could have one more celebration of our life together.

In earlier years we had always found fun ways to celebrate this day, such as planning a getaway to our Montana cabin or taking the ferry to Victoria, Canada. In more recent years, of course, the celebrations had become simpler but still meaningful: a favorite dinner at home, a special dessert, a nostalgic look at our wedding pictures and early to bed.

I knew that this particular anniversary would be our last and I wanted to make it special, but how could that be with Mike so ill; he could no longer eat by himself, speak, or move on his own. Life at this point in the illness had become so difficult for him, and for me.

But—and this is the most important point—I knew Mike was still there. He could still put his hand on mine, still pucker his lips for a kiss, and still look knowingly into my eyes. Yes, Mike was still here, and we were still in love. So how could we make our 45th anniversary a special day?

Gradually an idea formed in my mind: Mike always liked a little adventure. If he and I could somehow get out of the house and take a car ride together and perhaps buy some fresh flowers and Mike's favorite mocha drink—that would be lovely. However, first things first: I would need to get him safely out of bed and into the car which, at this point, would surely offer its own set of challenges.

OUR ADVENTURE BEGINS

Mike had a reasonable night's sleep, so the morning of our anniversary got off to a good start. With Mike doing his best to cooperate, I managed breakfast in bed, a bed bath, and clean clothes. I didn't mention our anniversary to him yet because, at this point, it would have been confusing to him and only slowed down our tasks. But Mike did seem to sense my happiness and we moved through the morning routine a little easier than some days.

Now the first challenge—could we make the transfer from his bed to the wheelchair? I say 'we' because I needed help from Mike and the Sit-to-Stand lift. We did it!

Mike was already in the wheelchair when Carol, our treasured weekly volunteer, arrived at 11:00 a.m. I asked if she thought we could get Mike into the car. It was something we had done together in the past, but each time it had become a little more difficult. "I'm willing to try," she said.

Next I asked Mike if he would like to go for a ride and he gave me a nod which meant yes. Not surprising, as Mike loved to be out and about. So now all three of us were up for the day's adventure.

The transfer into the car would be tricky. The challenge was for Mike to stand next to the open door with the window down. He needed to hold onto the doorframe, while Carol and I removed the wheelchair and rotated him into the seat. We only needed Mike to stand for a moment, but that might be too much for him. I could feel myself tense as we prepared for the big move and wondered: "45th anniversary or not, was I pushing the limit too far?" Fortunately, I spotted big, strong Julio the landscaper working in the yard next door, and he gladly helped us complete the mission.

Done! Mike was once again in the passenger seat, just like earlier days of the illness. It felt almost normal again. There was Mike, slouched happily in his seat with a cozy handmade shawl around his shoulders and his favorite derby hat on his head. Carol was in the back seat and I took the wheel, a little distracted perhaps by Carol's bubbly conversation, but, with one eye on Mike, I pressed the pedal and we were off!

In the back of my mind, I wondered how we would ever get Mike back into the house at the end of our outing, but we would cross that bridge when we came to it. For now, we would stick with the plan, because it all seemed so worthwhile.

And it *was* worthwhile! The ride to Bainbridge Gardens, our favorite nursery, was lovely. The sun shone through the tree branches, and the blackberry bushes showed their first flowers of the season. For this brief moment in time, we felt carefree and happy: all seemed well and almost normal, a touch of how it felt in years gone by, a nice ride with my husband Mike on a gorgeous spring day.

HUCKLEBERRY SHAKES

Following my plan for our little 45th wedding anniversary celebration, I parked at Bainbridge Gardens and told Carol and Mike that I would be right back. I scurried to the outdoor café, ordered two huckleberry milkshakes and delivered them to Mike and Carol in the car. Montana boys like their huckleberries!

While I headed back to the nursery to find a hanging fuchsia, Carol treated Mike to spoonfuls of milkshake. When I returned with the fuchsia, I traded roles with Carol, savoring the moment with my husband. True, it was hard for him to swallow, and little sips were all he could really handle, and there were soon milkshake drips everywhere (more napkins, Carol!) But I could tell Mike was glad to be out with his wife and helper, having this little treat, and enjoying the sunshine on his body as he sat with his legs out the door of the car.

It would have been wonderful to stay a little longer or go for an extended drive on the island, but I knew the eventual transfer to Mike's wheelchair at home would not be easy. It was time to head back. We all enjoyed the short ride home, but I could feel my shoulders tense as we neared the house. Always in the back of my mind was safety: will Mike or his caregivers get hurt? I knew that moving him by ourselves would be tricky, at best, and wished we had help.

As we pulled up to the house—yes!—there was Julio, still working in the garden and willing to help us again. Instead of moving Michael to the wheelchair, Julio swept him into his big arms like a small child and carried him right to the bedroom.

That touched me. It was heartbreaking to see this big strong healthy man carrying my small fragile husband in his arms. My tears flowed, knowing full well that this was truly "the last"—the last ride, the last time for Mike to be out in the world, and the last anniversary we would ever celebrate together. It sunk into me then: I was losing Michael and there was nothing I could do about it.

Sometimes your body encounters overwhelming sadness, and this was one of those times. You can keep that kind of sadness under wraps for only so long, and then it all comes out. It seems like the tears are too much at the time, but they are not, for these are the deep-down tears that have never been shed and need to come tumbling out.

Here was Julio, with tears of his own, gently laying Michael down on our bed. When I got to Michael's side, I fell to my knees, put my arms around him, and we cried together. We were both so vulnerable, both feeling the overwhelming realization and grief that soon it would all end. We could do no more, now, but we had both done our best. That moment was hopelessly sad but tender; I will always remember the feeling.

Carol and Julio departed with their own hearts filled with emotions, for they, too, had been immersed in that impossibly raw and moving moment in time.

HERE WE WERE ON THE FINAL MILE

Alone again, Mike and I cried together. And then I talked to him softly about our special day: "Mike, we had a nice ride, didn't we? Today is a beautiful day. I am glad we got out. Let me help you get comfortable. Julio helped us."

I'm not certain what else I said to Mike that day, but I know what was usually said. I would tell Mike, "Honey, it is really hard right now, but we are doing it. You are doing such a good job. You are still with me in our home—that was our plan and we are doing it."

I could feel our tension ease as I talked, and as he listened. Then I announced, "We have been married 45 years today, honey—happy anniversary!"

Despite all that Alzheimer's had thrown at us over the years, Mike and I had never let the disease pull us apart; instead we had turned to each other and pulled together. And here we were on the final mile of the journey, still traveling the road of life, still "Mike and Me" together through good times and hard. In that, we could both take pride.

Later that afternoon, we had a wonderful surprise! A dear friend and her young daughter came by with a beautiful anniversary cake, such a treat. She is a baker by profession, so this was not just any anniversary cake, it was lovingly prepared and so yummy, just the treat I needed! We have photos of the moment that clearly show Mike was indeed quite present and quite pleased to have both the company and the cake! It seemed that he was now aware that this was indeed a special day.

If I had to do that day all over again, would I? Absolutely! Our anniversary adventure had not been easy, but then none of the last days were. There had been 44 other anniversaries over the years, complete with flowers, dinners out, date nights, or romantic trips away, but none are remembered as fondly as our 45th.

Looking back, I think Mike in his own way was glad we went. I think he enjoyed the adventure. I think he appreciated his milkshake and the cake and the hugs at the end of the day. I do know he would be proud that he did it for me. It was a gift he gave me, one last outing filled with memories for me that I will always and forever cherish.

INSIGHTS

- Early in the illness someone counseled me to keep things as "normal" as possible as long as possible—such good advice! it was one of the golden rules Mike and I lived by on our Alzheimer's journey–and so I am passing that same counsel on to you again here.

- Why bother to plan an anniversary outing with someone who can no longer walk, talk or remember? Because having an anniversary celebration had been a tradition for 44 years. Keeping that special celebration right up to the end made a difference. It affirmed our semi-independence from Alzheimer's and gave me something to look forward to—a day to make a plan for something special in our lives.

- It was a special day for Mike too; he got to be out of the house, seeing the world, listening to the birds, hearing the laughter, feeling the sun, and experiencing the love of his wife.

- I invite you to do the same. Despite Alzheimer's, my wish is for you and your loved one to live each day to the fullest, and to decide to keep your life as normal as possible as long as possible. You will be glad that you did not let the "lasts" enter your life before it was absolutely necessary.

- Keep marking dates and events on your calendar. Give yourself and your loved one something to look forward to. Create fun! Live with the anticipation of something wonderful still around the corner. You both deserve it.

- Not everyone will choose to stretch it as far as I did, with an outdoor adventure in the car so close to the end. Your stretch might be to simply invite a friend in for a cup of tea and ask them to bring a treat, or pick a special movie to watch at home, or have a huge bouquet of flowers delivered, or buy meaningful music to play. Whatever it is, celebrate your special day; do it for you and for the person you love.

- Don't listen to the well-intentioned naysayers who may lovingly advise you to give up your old celebrations or traditions. Despite Alzheimer's, you will be surprised by what you can continue to do and how long you can do it. Get your friends and family involved, they can help you keep living, dreaming and enjoying your lives to the very end—just as it was meant to be.

- Keep making memories as long as you can. The loved one with Alzheimer's will enjoy the "moment" and you and those who surround you will enjoy the "memory." People seldom regret the memories they create; they only regret the moments they did *not* have.

PART XI

~

Accepting that the
End of Life is Near

WHEN HOSPICE JOINED OUR CIRCLE

*I suspected we might be nearing the
time for hospice, but suddenly it
was right in front of us—
and I didn't like it.*

EIGHT-AND-A-HALF YEARS AFTER DR. JUNG informed us that
Mike had Alzheimer's, there came another day I will never forget.
Mike and I were sitting together in Dr. Jung's exam room. She listened, as always, as we told her how much the disease had progressed over the past few months. Finally, she looked up and said
gently, "It might be time for Mike to enter the hospice program."

How could we ever reconcile the choice we now had to make:
on the one hand we knew that hospice would offer the kind of added help we now urgently needed for Mike; on the other hand, it
also felt like we would be surrendering hope that Mike would ever
get better. On top of which was the question of whether or not we
were willing to have hospice enter our close-knit circle of friends
and family.

Over the next week or so, Mike and I had time to settle into the
idea of hospice care. We even convinced ourselves that we were ready
to meet in our home with the hospice nurse, but we really weren't.

MEETING WITH HOSPICE

I will never forget the day hospice came to our home to evaluate
Mike. There had been other hard days, but not quite like this. I got
the house picked up before our appointment, but that's about all I

had time to do. Mike was clean and tidy with a fresh pullover shirt, and I had cookies handy if it seemed like they should be offered.

The day itself was beautiful, a sunny warm August day, a day Mike and I had anticipated but also dreaded—a day we would sit on the deck to talk to the people from hospice.

Soon two nice ladies arrived at our door—a social worker and a nurse. Mike and I immediately liked them both; we just didn't like what we were about to discuss with them.

I offered tea and cookies. We sipped and they assessed. Could Mike hold the cup by himself? How much help did he need at this point? Would he mind walking across the deck (which he did with me close behind, no falls—not now). He walked sideways, not straight ahead, for that was the best he could do. They praised him, and they assessed him.

Next came questions about life skills: did Mike need help eating?...yes...dressing?...yes...help in the bathroom?...yes. I felt conflicted. I wondered what the right answers should be. I instinctively wanted to tell them how well Mike was doing and I did, but was that the wrong thing to tell hospice? Shouldn't I be telling hospice all the things he could no longer do? I wanted my husband to "pass" this assessment so he could be approved for hospice—or did I?

Finally the assessment was finished and Mike and I were told that he had "qualified" for hospice. We listened to all the services that hospice could offer: a nurse's aid to help with a shower, his nails, and bedding once a week—wonderful! A massage therapist every other week. A social worker and a chaplin, and weekly visits by a home healthcare nurse. All great news!

But then came the paradox of hospice care: in order for Mike to continue to qualify for all this assistance, he could not get better or show improvement. In other words, Mike had to continue to go downhill to stay in the program. After nearly nine years of hoping and praying for a cure, it didn't feel right to give up on getting better. That was just so hard to accept and brought tears to my eyes.

The hospice ladies asked if I had Mike's power of attorney and wanted to see the documents. I knew right where they were, but I did not want to leave Mike alone even for a minute with two strangers. Yes, they were nice people, but I was his protector, and they couldn't possibly understand all that my husband might need. Finally, I told Mike I would be right back with the papers and returned quickly.

With the documents laid out on the table it was time to once again look at the life choices Mike had made so long ago, including no IVs, no tube feeding, and no extraordinary measures. All were in line with the requirements of hospice.

Now, I turned to Mike to be sure he wanted me to sign the hospice papers. We had talked about all this before, but still I wanted to ask him one more time. Is this what you want? Once again, I explained as clearly as I could what we were doing and what it would mean to both of us. I assured him that it seemed like the best choice to me, but I asked again, "Mike, is this what you want to do?"

There was a great deal of crying that day on my part and Mike's. If I had been able to hold it together I know it would have been such a comfort to Mike, and yet I could not. The caring social worker and nurse sat quietly and let our decision slowly unfold, for they had done this before, and we had not.

This was not about the nurse or caring social worker; it was about us—Mike and me—and his ultimate life choice. Finally, Mike gave me a nod and I knew it was his way of telling me to sign the papers. I signed the multiple documents, including one that said that Mike was not to be resuscitated.

That was so difficult! For now we were basically saying that there is no way out of this except Mike's death. I was simply not prepared to give up hope. Hope had been our oxygen supply. Looking forward to a new breakthrough or a miracle cure had always been such an integral part of how we approached the journey. But now a "no resuscitation" sign on our refrigerator felt ... well, hopeless.

At some point the hospice nurse and social worker did assure us that if Mike somehow got better then he could simply withdraw from hospice, and that sometimes happened. I liked having that sliver of hope. And so we took a deep breath, dried our eyes, and pulled out the insurance and Medicare cards to make it official.

The hospice nurse then asked if she could give Mike a physical assessment and we walked sideways into the bedroom. This was the easy part: blood pressure, pulse, and a few more questions. This would now be the baseline they would work from in the future.

PRAISE FOR HOSPICE

If I sound a little hostile, please know that my hostility is aimed at Alzheimer's not at hospice. Truly, the entire hospice staff was wonderful to Mike and me and our family. Hospice entered our circle in August and they provided all they promised and more, including the physical and emotional support that Mike and I truly needed the last ten months of his life.

By the way, there was a brief but wonderful period in those last few months where Mike had a little bounce and started doing better. We had no idea why, but he was talking and moving around a little better. The nurse even said that if this improvement continued he might have to leave the program. There was that hospice paradox again: the nurse had to show on her assessments that Mike was declining, while at the same time I was still hoping and praying he would rebound completely.

As it turned out his little bounce did not last long, so he continued to pass hospice with flying colors—darn!

(See my hospice journal notes next page)

AUGUST 4

Mike went into hospice care today.
It was strange making this decision official—no more life-saving
measures. He is still so with me it is hard to think of giving him up.
I know this is what he wants, but there is such a switch from
working toward wellness to palliative care.

Should I continue to work on him walking?
Does he get his teeth cleaned or go to the dentist anymore?
Hospice tells me it is no longer necessary for him to go to the doctor.
They will give weekly reports.

AUGUST 14

Having Mike in hospice has changed the focus from how to deal
with Alzheimer's to how to prepare for death. I am oh-so-not ready
for this change. I don't want Mike to die. He has been with me for
so very long, I don't want to be without him.

~

Even in hospice, our life is filled with purpose and meaning. Our
days are simple, but they are still our life: Sit on the deck and
watch the boats. Or Mike sits in a deck chair in the driveway while
I water. Our daily walk to the mailbox. A ride into town. Mike
usually stays in the car, the aisles are too small for his wheelchair. I
get coffee from Rolling Bay and we go to Fay Bainbridge Park.

~

Tonight we watered the plants for Kathleen and Sam. Mike saw
the moon and pointed to it. He was so pleased. I said,
"Moon, say moon." He did, but I think it changed the
specialness of his showing me.

While at Kathleen and Sam's he leaned over in the car to give me a
kiss. I love him so very much, I am not ready to say goodbye.

SEPTEMBER 9

*I went to Hospice House. If there is room available, then Mike can
stay five days at Hospice House. But, now is not the time to leave
him. I actually want more time with him. Lots of help is needed,
but that means less time for us together. He still misses me when
I am gone, and I miss him.*

INSIGHTS

- Even in the final months Mike still recognized me and knew me, which was something I did not expect. After all, I had been told that he would likely be in a full-time care facility by now.

- Allowing hospice to join our circle of friends and family made it possible for Mike and me to stay together in our home. We were still working with our original plan from eight-and-a-half years earlier: *Keep Mike at home as long as possible.*

- You might wonder why I asked Mike if he wanted to sign the hospice papers even though I had his power of attorney. I sought his okay because he was still physically and emotionally present and still my husband. We were talking about his life and he deserved the dignity of participating in the decisions. If he had told me no, I would have told the hospice ladies we were not ready to sign today.

- People with Alzheimer's deserve all the dignity we can give them, perhaps more than the average person, for it is hard for them to come by it.

- At first we did not like the idea of hospice people coming and going in our home, but soon we looked forward to the hospice visits and were disappointed if someone had to cancel.

- I learned that while hospice did not give us hope for a cure, they provided a different kind of hope: hope for no pain, hope for a nice day, hope for dignity with death, and hope for meaning to the very end of one's life.

- I recently heard that the words "Do Not Resuscitate" are now often replaced by "Allow Natural Death." That wording would have been so much easier to accept.

- It seems that signing hospice papers is difficult for everyone. Perhaps the best you can do is to be prepared for it. You do want the help and on some level you do want this illness to end, but actually accepting you are ready to die or have your loved one die is a different matter.

- Just remember, you are not alone. Your circle of friends and family are with you at the end, just as they were all along.

DISCUSSING LIFE AND DEATH

My hope for you and your loved one
is that you do not fear the end of life
conversations when they arrive.

THE DECISION TO BRING HOSPICE into our home had been
huge. It meant that our long-standing hope for a last-minute cure
had now been formally replaced by the acknowledgment that
Mike's life was, in fact, coming to a close. And yet, while Mike and I
had made the hospice decision together, neither one of us was prepared at this point to fully accept or discuss what it meant.

Over our 40 plus years of marriage, Mike and I had spoken here
and there of death and dying. Early in his illness we had also discussed what he wanted at the end of life—and even imagined what
the final days might be like with Alzheimer's. However, when your
loved one is actually nearing his or her time, it just feels like a different kind of conversation is needed. Even more challenging, how do
you carry on that conversation when the person you are speaking
with has limited ability to talk or reason?

I can't claim to have the answers, but I do know what worked
for Mike and me. For starters, I did not try to sit down with Mike
and have a big "death and dying conversation" all at once. But I did
decide that I would no longer avoid the "D" word; in fact, I would
look for ways to broach the subject when Mike seemed open to it.

Gradually, I began to realize that those open moments
came when Mike was upset and crying for no obvious reason.
At these times it just felt to me that he was trying to tell me
that he did not want to die. I tried to verbalize the words he

was struggling with to let him know that I understood what he was feeling. When I got it right he would calm immediately and I knew that I had put my finger on his fears. At that point we often held each other and cried together.

I didn't realize it at the time, but each of those little moments of mutual sadness and grief were moving us closer and closer to accepting the inevitability of his death.

~ FROM MY JOURNAL ~
AUGUST (YEAR 9)

We had a lovely tender moment at St. B's with Father Dennis. I became tearful and Mike looked at me with all the love he has always had for me. His hand reached out, and he began to cry with me. I went over to his side, sat on the floor next to his chair and put my arm around him. I told him it was okay to cry. It was just getting hard now. But we still had much to be grateful for—we still have our good moments.

NOVEMBER (YEAR 9)

Mike and I had a nice moment on Thursday. We were in the kitchen and he began to cry as he told me "I love you." I put my arms around him and said "I love you too" as we cried together. I also said. "It is hard now, but we are doing it—we are a good team. No one knows when they will die or go to heaven. I am not ready for you to go yet. It is not time yet."

Then I said: "We will know when it is time. You let me know when you are ready. I hope I am ready when you want to go." The cry and the talk helped us both. We blew our noses and moved into dinner feeling better.

(continued on next page)

DECEMBER (YEAR 9)

Once again Mike began to cry at lunchtime. I asked why he was crying. "Is it because you are going to die?" I got a nod. I told him we don't know when we will die, but you are not getting better and Dr. Jung has nothing else we can do. More tears!

But, we have done everything we need to do, including: Power of Attorney... deciding how you want to die... staying here in our home... and no IVs or feeding tubes.

(Sister) Patty has been staying with us. She wonders if Mike is done living now. I need to ask Mike. If so, I need to let him know that I am now ready to let him go.

On January 16, three-and-a-half months before Mike died, I sat on the couch with him and held his hand. I told him I did not think it was time for him to die, but whenever he was ready, I was now ready too.

I assured him that when it became too hard for him, he could let go and I would be okay. There were lots of tears and I-love-yous but there was no anger or fear, just a calm acceptance. In some ways that moment seems like it was our first real goodbye.

─────────────── **INSIGHTS** ───────────────

- Over our many years of marriage Mike and I had many important conversations, and yet we almost missed one of the most important conversations of all. As the time for Mike to depart neared, his speech was so limited that it was nearly impossible to communicate. And yet with his tears and nods and touches, I knew just what he was telling me. He still loved life and he still loved me and did not want to die.

- Gradually, each of those little conversations that were filled with tears and nods moved us ever closer to accepting that soon Mike and I would no longer be together in the life we had known for more than 40 years. They were painful moments at the time but I look back on them as some of the most meaningful and courageous of our life together.

- My hope for you and your loved one is that you not fear these conversations when they arrive. They are usually not planned, they simply happen. The most I could do at the time was to accept and not fear them—to remain present and not run away from them—for at those moments I had the privilege of entering Mike's world as he moved a little closer to the mystery of life and death.

- Atul Gawande's book <u>Being Mortal</u> tells us the importance of talking about death and dying with the one we love and gives us insight into how we can talk about this difficult subject. I recommend it.

- Thanks to our mutual faith and prayers, along with our multiple little talks over time, I believe that when it was time for Mike to die, he was at peace—something we all want when our time comes.

CHAPTER 48

MIKE'S LAST VISIT TO DR. JUNG

*Clear advice and calming words
near the end of the journey from our
beloved doctor.*

IT WAS DECEMBER AND MIKE HAD BEEN under hospice care for the past four months. But he was still scheduled for an appointment with Dr. Jung. Under the circumstances, I wondered if we should cancel that appointment. Such a debate: since we are in hospice, now, should we go to our doctor one last time or not? It would be a difficult trip to her Seattle office with Mike so ill, but I finally decided we should go.

Over the previous nine years, Dr. Jung had accompanied Mike and me on every step of our journey through Alzheimer's. Along the way she had shared our dreams, calmed our fears, encouraged our experiments, and celebrated our ongoing vacations, adventures and family milestones.

At each appointment she had a way of gently moving us forward and alerting us about what would come next. I wondered how she could possibly help us at this final visit to her office.

On the morning of our appointment I had everything ready to make the trip as easy as possible for Mike: his clothes were laid out, extra blankets for the car, water bottle, and CDs. Betty, our hospice aide, would arrive early and help me get Mike bathed, dressed, and safely in the car. Our son Patrick, who was home for winter break, would meet us on the waterfront when we drove off the ferry and would go up the hill with us to Swedish Medical Center.

All hinged on how the morning went with Mike. At that point in his illness we usually awakened a few times during the night, but this particular night had been restful so that was good. Nevertheless, in the morning it was raining and things began to fall apart.

Mike woke tearful and agitated. We got through breakfast, but first lots of tears. I heard him say "die." I asked, are you talking about dying? "Yes, I'm dying." As I cried I told him yes he was dying. It was like saying there is no more Santa. I had been going around not saying the words and now they were said. Mike's response was: "I don't want to die."

I repeated his words and he began to cry harder. "I'm going to die." He cried and we cried together. There was lots of crying and some yelling. I softened it by saying, "We always have hope." I told him, "I don't want you to go."

Lots more crying, but he settled when I said, "We are going to see Dr. Jung today. Do you want to see Dr. Jung?" He shook his head yes. "Okay, let's get ready." I gave him half a Lorazepam pill behind his lip to relax him so Betty and I could get him ready.

Now Betty arrived and helped me do a quick bed bath, for we were now under a time crunch. We needed to get Mike in the car before the Lorazepam made him too sleepy for the move. On with his pullover shirt, pullup pants, maroon jacket with easy zipper, and into the wheelchair.

Mike was no longer yelling, he was fully awake and cooperating in every way with two ladies who were rapidly dressing him in time to catch the next ferry.

Thanks to Betty, the transfer from home to car went well. Pat met us on the waterfront and the transfer from car to hospital/doctor's

office went well, too, with a mocha en route. Patrick gave Mike a
walk around the hall, but Mike was exhausted and ultimately slept
through Dr. Jung's visit.

~

Dr. Jung was wonderful as usual. She talked about death with
Alzheimer's: "It is not painful, and I can help you with medication
if necessary. Your brain and body slow and you just go to sleep. No
advantage in extending life with tube feedings or IV. I will help in
any way I can. Mike does not need to suffer. She went on to say, "It
is now about you, Rosalys. You need to take care of yourself." We
hugged and said our farewell, as this will be our last doctor's visit.
Patrick returned to the island with us, which was helpful.

As always, Dr. Jung had listened carefully and then said all the right
things. I had some tears while she talked, but not like the cry I had
with Mike earlier. I knew I needed to hear what Dr. Jung was saying
and absorb what we could expect next.

Mike had slept through most of the visit. It was now late in the
day and we had missed his time of clarity. Perhaps the great gift for
Mike that day was having a mocha and a walk around the hall with
his son. I was surprised that Mike was able to walk that day, but he
always did the best he could for his son.

I was sorry Mike could not be more present and yet maybe it was
just how it was meant to be. This final doctor's appointment had
really helped me. Dr. Jung's calm manner, clear advice, and caring
words were just what I needed.

The following journal note, written a day after our last visit with
Dr. Jung, is a reminder of how much I continued to love Mike every
step of the way. And how I was able to manage our journey together
by looking for the silver lining in every situation. My philosophy
was simply to do what I could and then live in the moment and
enjoy all that remained for us. For, despite Alzheimer's, we still had
much to be thankful for.

Mike awoke this morning agitated. I turned to him and talked about our life story, and he settled. Oh how I continue to love Mike. He is so responsive to me. It is like when we began to date. It is all about us and our love for each other. If we go from this closeness to death it will be very difficult.

~

I awoke a few days ago feeling that Mike had died. The physical feeling was so overwhelming. It's one I have felt several times before and do not like: Mama, Daddy, Grandma. I am so glad no Getaway Weekend classes for awhile, I want my time with Mike.

INSIGHTS

- Dr. Jung was such a gift to Mike and me. She was with us in spirit and, in fact, during every step of our Alzheimer's journey. You and your loved one need and deserve this kind of caring relationship with your primary doctor. If you don't have it, I highly recommend you consider finding another doctor.

- It may sound surprising, but even in our last seven months together Mike and I were still very emotionally connected and present with each other. As hard as some days could be, I did not want it to end. We were never so much in love. Alzheimer's had not taken that away.

- After that final visit, I did not need to rely on Dr. Jung to assess medication or help with Mike's care because hospice was now there for our daily needs.

- Even when Mike could no longer say the words, our little talks together were still important. Now I needed to say the words for him so he would know I understood what he was trying to say. Now he was trying to tell me, "I know I am going to die." I had to accept and acknowledge that stark sentence by telling him I heard him and understood.

- Around this time the social worker from hospice told me that things would not get more difficult than they were right now. That was helpful because I was uncertain if I could handle "harder." And she was right. The last few months became easier because Mike slept more and became calmer.

- There was one more reason why I decided to take Mike to that final doctor's appointment with Dr. Jung: because he wanted to go. Even at that advanced stage in his illness, I felt it was important that he remain in charge of anything that he could be in charge of. When I asked Mike if he wanted to go to Dr. Jung's, he said yes, so we went.

- Here are the gifts our last doctor's appointment brought to us: Mike got out of the house, had a ferry ride, a mocha, had time with his son, and saw Dr. Jung one last time. Dr. Jung also got to say goodbye. I learned what would come next and got the support I needed. Patrick, too, learned what would come next and had an important moment in time with his dad.

- Though we were nearing the end, this was still Mike's life and those who loved him were here to support him in any way, just as he would have done for us if the situation were reversed.

CHAPTER 49

WHAT OUR LAST FEW MONTHS TOGETHER WERE LIKE

*Throughout the final year I focused
on gratitude for the days that
remained and which continued to be
filled with love and tenderness.*

NEW YEAR'S DAY OF MIKE'S TENTH YEAR rolled around and, despite all the ups and downs we had experienced through the years of his illness, we were still sharing life together in our home. I did not know what would lie ahead for us that year; I was just hoping against hope that I could continue giving Mike the love and support he would need to spend his final chapter at home.

Our last months together were astonishing in some ways, and filled with memories that I now treasure. On one level our daily life had become so difficult, and yet so loving and tender on another. Here we were—nearly a decade after his diagnosis—still in love, still finding ways to communicate, but now experiencing the impending mystery of life and death.

At this point in the journey Mike needed more help with the most basic life skills such as dressing, sitting and eating. Early in that year he could only walk a few steps on his own, and later not at all. At that time I had not yet discovered the Sit-to-Stand machine, so the most difficult tasks for me at the beginning of year 10 were getting him in and out of bed or in and out of the car. If I did not have help, I could no longer get him safely up or out and about in the world, and this made a huge difference in his day and mine.

Mike's occasional outbursts seemed to escalate in January and February, then gradually decreased and finally stopped altogether. I sometimes saw tears in his eyes which made me cry too. And there were conversations about facing and accepting death right up to the very end—and those were never easy for me or for him.

Life in that final year was a roller-coaster ride of ups and downs—good days and bad days—and that's part of what made it so emotionally draining. When a good day would come, it gave me hope that Mike was possibly getting better and that more good days might follow. And then a hard day would come, and that always made me fear that this was going to be the new norm.

This may be difficult for some people to accept but, on an emotional level, the Mike I had always known and loved was still there in the final months, still reaching out to me. Sometimes he was uncertain of who I was and that, too, brought tears to my eyes, but with a simple 'clink' of our wedding rings and a little eye-to-eye conversation he could come back to me.

FOCUSING ON GRATITUDE

At night, my sleep was becoming more and more fitful. My dreams increased and were sometimes dark, waking me with a panicked feeling that Mike had died. Then there was the night I dreamed of all the good things—our first date, anniversaries, weddings, births, lovemaking, laughter, Mountain Brook, and working together in the yard, all rolled into one. That dream gave me hope that my happy memories would somehow remain.

Throughout the final year I could not allow myself to dwell on how difficult life had become for Mike and me. Instead I focused on feelings of gratitude for the days that remained and which continued to be filled with love and tenderness. I was in constant conflict. I did not want my time with my dear husband to end, but I did not want him to suffer either. And, as always, I continued to wonder, "Can I do this?"

One day a hospice nurse came to our home and surprised me by saying, "You are still making memories." I had not thought of that. She was right—these difficult last months were still part of our life-long love story and, regardless of the difficulty, I wanted to be fully present with Mike for this last chapter.

The next day, I got the camera out and started taking photos that are now priceless to me: I took photos of our last outings together; of our 45th wedding anniversary on May 21st; of Mike's seventy-sixth birthday on May 23rd; of Kathleen, Pat, and me sitting on Mike's bed with him; of Mike and me holding hands with our wedding rings; and of Riley's tea parties and tents in our room.

I took photos, too, of our special helpers who would soon come to our home no more. And I must say that in all these 'end of life' photos, Mike looks quite content surrounded by those he loved.

OUR CONVERSATIONS NEVER STOPPED

In the late stages of Alzheimer's, when your loved one has almost certainly lost the ability to speak, it's easy to conclude that he or she is no longer there—but that was not the case for Mike and me.

I always felt that Mike was still present, so I continued to converse with him as if he were. True, there were times when I was uncertain if Mike still knew me, but then later he would show me that he did, so I never gave up on talking to him. And the reward was that he never gave up on trying to communicate with me either.

In January my sister Patty and I went away for two nights. As usual, I told Mike where I was going and when I would return. When I came home two days later, however, Mike at first gave me no facial indication that he even knew I had been gone. That night I feared that he would know me no more, but that was not the case. The next morning he greeted me with, "Where, Why, You?" He was clearly asking me where I had been and what I had been up to. In the final stages of Alzheimer's, those three words from my husband and friend certainly counted as a bona fide conversation with me.

JANUARY 9
Last night I felt tearful after book club. I told Wendy as I had told Kathleen that I was glad to hear Sabina say that some (Alzheimer's patients) continue living at this level for a year. I am still not ready to say goodbye.

MARCH 22
No more tears. Some yelling but it no longer scares me.
He settles so easy when I change activity.
Sleep is the biggest challenge. If I can get a chunk of 3–4 hours, then I am happy. Mike sleeps about 1½ to 2 hours usually.

Stephanie was here today; we got Mike (in wheelchair) and Riley out for a walk. Stopped and talked with our neighbor Matt while he prepared his garden.

I need to ask Mike if he is ready to die.
I need to have Father Dennis come for a visit.

APRIL 3
A couple of weeks ago I asked Mike if he was ready to die—he told me "no." I told him I didn't want him to go, but when it was time I was ready.

~

Mike was tearful when I returned from work on Sunday. I said it is okay for us to cry—-this is sad and hard. Alzheimer's is not easy, we knew it would get hard and it is hard now. When you need to die I understand and I will be okay. You have taken good care of your family. I love you. If you die before me, and it looks like you will, keep a place for me because I will be coming to join you. I told him some people are not so lucky to have loved someone. We are very lucky. We have been married 44 years. Once again I tapped our rings and showed him "We go together."

APRIL 6

Before I left for Swedish Hospital, yesterday, I told Mike I would miss him. He didn't seem to get what I was saying. I explained I had to go to work, but would miss him. I continued to fix lunch. When I looked back he was crying. I asked if it was because he would miss me too—he nodded yes. We are still connected.

APRIL 12

Yesterday after breakfast Mike began to cry silent tears, and he and I had our little visit as we sometimes do about death.

"What is wrong? Are you sad? Do you have pain? Are you thinking about dying?"

"No one knows when they will die, but we are all going to die . . . you have Alzheimer's and we cannot get you better. We have done everything we can. I don't want you to die, but when you think it is time and have to go, I will be okay. You have taken good care of Patrick, Kathleen and me. I will be all right."

Mike continued to cry, but was not upset like sometimes when we talk. No crying out this time. He then shook his head, sniffed, and stopped crying. I could tell he was saying "enough of this."

I asked, "are you okay, are you done crying—is this enough of this?" I clearly got the sense that that was what he was telling me.

I told him that I loved him and that we still had some time together.

MAY 1

We have a beautiful sunny day today. I am sitting in the bedroom with the window open, the sun is coming in, Mike is awake and cleaned up, listening to birds, airplane, and children. It is wonderful.

I am ready for summer; I think I missed spring. Time to share the photo album with Mike.

THE MYSTERIES OF LIFE AND DEATH

When death is near, there is a time of preparation that is often beyond our understanding. The dying sometimes report experiencing a light they cannot explain or seeing people no one else can see.

In the last months leading up to Mike's death, he would sometimes point out the window or at the corner of the room and ask if I could see someone. I could not, but I never had the feeling that he was simply out of his mind. He seemed clearheaded at the time, undisturbed by the event, sometimes even smiling, and he was surprised that I did not see the people he showed me. I never agreed or disagreed with him, I just explained that I did not see them.

⟶ FROM MY JOURNAL ⟵
JANUARY 20

One night at bedtime while Mike sat on the side of the bed he pointed toward the chair, "her, her, her." I asked, "What do you see, do you see a woman?" He answered yes. "Is it your mother or granny?" I asked. "No" —he gave me a funny look like I was crazy thinking it could be Granny or his mother. When I settled him in bed, I said I wondered if it could be an angel.
He calmed and went to sleep.

While on a car picnic at Fay Bainbridge Park I again talked about angels. Mike was very clear-minded at the time. I asked him, "Do you believe in angels?" "No" and he gave me a cute look.
I said I do and that some people see them when they are sick.
"I wonder if you have been seeing angels? Sometimes you see people I don't see."

He said "You, you, you, are my angel."

We began to cry as I talked about how we always knew this would get hard and it is now. I talked about all the good times we had during the previous years of Alzheimer's and how much I loved him.

- Author Libby Fudim wrote, "Recall as often as you want. A happy memory never wears out." It's true. I'm sure I will never fully forget the hard times Mike and I experienced. But it's the happy memories that I now hold dear and recall again and again. Memories of our amazing friends and family who helped us along the way, of our quiet afternoon naps, our conversations, our smiles, our commitment to each other and the wonderful life we made, despite the shadow of Alzheimer's.

- During those last months Mike wanted me by his side as much as possible. Music, stories on CDs or movies worked for a time, but toward the end there was no substitute for our being together.

- Some Alzheimer's couples move the hospital bed to the living room to allow their loved one to always be with the family. Mike and I preferred to maintain our quiet bedroom space that was sometimes reserved only for us. This meant getting Mike out of bed and into the living room each day, but it was worth it.

- In the final year I moved my journal to the shelf next to the bed so I would write more often and made a special point to capture the joyful moments along the way, of which there were many. Example: *January 1—Lunch at Art and Wendy's—Mike gave a salute when he saw Art's photo in uniform; Mike looked up from his wheelchair and saw his graduation photo on the wall and said, "That is me." I got Mike in and out of the car by myself today—with the help of the door. We went out for pizza!*

- Whenever Mike was sad and tearful during this time, I did not disregard his feelings or try to make them go away. I simply tried to understand how hard this was for him. Understanding his feelings was one gift I could give him. As Mike's sadness eased, I often talked of a more pleasant memory and told him what a good job we were doing managing this difficult time.

- I continued to teach one day a week at the hospital right up until the last week of Mike's life. Why? Because, as hard as it was to leave Mike's side those last months, I knew I needed that day away to recharge my batteries so I could be at my best the rest of the time for Mike. I encourage you to consider doing something similar.

- I beat the odds and did not become sick or ill during Mike's illness. Let me remind you again of the wisdom of the emergency airline motto to "put your own oxygen mask on first." Only by remaining strong and healthy yourself can you then turn your attention to fully helping your loved one.

- Some have asked me how I managed to take this long, difficult journey with my husband up to the very last day. By now, I think you know the answer: I never could have done it alone. I was able to do it only because I had lots of help from our circle of family, friends and caregivers– and because I approached the Alzheimer's journey "one day at a time" so that it would not overwhelm me.

CHAPTER 50

KEEPING OUR MARRIAGE BED

Mike and I had been sleeping together
for 45 years, and we weren't
about to stop now.

MIKE AND I LIKED OUR BED. It was queen-sized and soft in all the right places. And it was not just for sleeping, it was our place to talk, snuggle, laugh and make love.

By the time hospice entered our life in year nine, our bed was no longer working for us the way it had in the past. We still liked to snuggle and have our intimate conversations at night, but the bed had a new job now. It was a place for Mike to eat his breakfast in the morning, a place I needed to move him into at night and out of in the morning—and a place for naps.

Breakfast in bed had become important because Mike had to eat before he could have his Alzheimer's medication. Then there was a predictable nap about an hour or so after his medication, which made him more capable of helping me transfer him out of bed later. So our daily routine was breakfast in bed, pills, a nap, and then the transfer.

Propping Mike up in our queen-sized bed for breakfast had become complicated. Even with all the right pillows in just the right places, he would slip into an uncomfortable slouch. I knew the answer was a hospital bed, but I resisted the idea of moving our "marriage bed" out.

One day when the social worker came to call, she insisted that it was now time to get a hospital bed, which triggered a heated discussion. It was like we were having two different conversations. She was talking about the value of having a safe bed at the right height, one that would put Mike in a sitting position. I, on the other hand, was talking about touch, cuddling, holding each other, being married and sleeping together for 45 years. We were not speaking the same language, yet I knew there was merit in what she was saying.

A PLAN TO KEEP US SLEEPING TOGETHER

I held out a week or so longer and then I finally called Tim's Home Medical Supply store to arrange for a hospital bed to be delivered. Before calling Tim's, however, I came up with a plan: if I moved the old twin bed from my home office and pushed it tightly against Mike's new hospital bed, maybe we could still be close and snuggle.

The next day I drove to Penney's Department Store and picked up the materials I needed to execute the plan, including twin mattress pads, sheets, blankets and—most important—a king-sized bed cover that would make the two little beds look like one big marriage bed. Done!

When the hospital bed arrived the next morning, I was ready. We moved the queen bed into the entryway for now. Then we pushed the hospital bed and the small twin from my office together.

The bedding worked perfectly. The twin sheets and blanket gave Mike his own easy-to-change bed, and my twin bed next to it could be pulled away when needed for access. The king cover made it look less like a hospital bed, and more like the same big queen that we had enjoyed for the past 45 years.

Recognizing the benefits of sleeping next to each other, even during the final period of hospice, is the main point of this chapter.

I still remember fondly our last nights in bed together. And, oh, our afternoon naps during Mike's last few weeks were so special. People would come and go, and then it was time for Mike and me to take our afternoon nap. I would close our bedroom door and we would snuggle close, sometimes have a little one-way chat, hold each other and fall into a peaceful sleep, just like we had for 45 years.

INSIGHTS

- Today, I wonder why hospital beds are not widely available in a larger size for two people. When you rent a hospital bed it would be lovely to be asked, "Would you like a twin or a double?"

- When it was time for the hospital bed to go back to the medical supply store, I discovered I had developed a love/hate relationship with it. It was surprisingly difficult to see it go. It had now become a part of our love story and our life together.

- Much is written about touch and the value it provides each of us, so it gets its own chapter next. For now, I simply say, sleeping next to Mike and being able to hold each other at night and during our afternoon nap was a treasured part of our last months, weeks, and days together.

- I slept close to Mike because I loved him and because I believe it made a difference for both of us. Perhaps someday there will be actual research verifying the emotional and medical advantages of sleeping close to the one you love who has Alzheimer's.

- I am thankful that we did not miss out on these last days of cuddling and sleeping together. As always, I am not suggesting that everyone should do as we did. I am simply telling the story so you and others will know that there is more than one way to spend your last days together.

CHAPTER 51

HUMAN TOUCH IS THERAPY

*I believe that loving touch made
a positive difference for Mike,
helping him stay connected to me
and extending both the length and
the quality of his life.*

BETTY, THE NURSE'S AIDE FROM HOSPICE who came to our house once a week, was knowledgeable and bighearted.

When helping me with Mike, Betty understood the power of little things—how a simple touch, a smile, a hug or the smallest act of caring or comforting could eliminate his stress and brighten his day. She was always willing to go along with what I thought best for Mike—be it a shower, a pedicure, a change of sheets, or a soothing hand massage. And the best part was that she always arrived with a positive attitude and a smile. We loved Betty.

Then one day, as we neared the final weeks of Mike's life, Betty offered something that I did not want. In her compassionate way she asked, "Would it be okay if I brought a doll for Mike to cuddle?" Such a kind offer from such a kind person, how could I possibly tell her no, but I did.

Diplomatically but firmly, I explained to Betty that Mike would not want a doll, that he never wanted a doll and would not want one now. "Besides," I explained, "Mike and I are still husband and wife, and we are still cuddling every night, so a doll will not be necessary."

That said, Betty and I both affirmed that even in the final weeks of Mike's Alzheimer's journey we would ensure that he was treated with dignity as my husband, including lots of human touch, loving hugs and soothing massage.

HUMAN TOUCH AS THERAPY

"Take someone's hand and you touch their heart," wrote Mother Teresa. Today's medical community would certainly agree. Pediatric researchers have known for a long time that skin-to-skin contact with babies is crucial to their healthy development and sense of well-being. A mother's consistent loving touch calms newborns and infants: they cry less and sleep better, and their brain and emotional development are also facilitated.

More recently, we have learned just how important human touch can be for adults too. We now know that touch can calm us in times of stress, decrease elevated blood pressure, ease depression, hasten healing, and increase overall longevity.

It's no surprise, then, that massage is becoming a recognized and accepted practice in mainstream medicine and is covered by conventional insurance and even offered to those in hospice care.

Knowing all of the above, I wondered if I could make a difference for Mike by simply maintaining the everyday touching, hugging and cuddling that we had shared for so many years. I thought so and was careful not to back away as the disease progressed. I vowed that his wheelchair, hospital bed, and sit-to-stand machine would not prevent Mike and me from continuing the tender human touch that we had always shared.

HOW TO KEEP 'IN TOUCH' WITH YOUR LOVED ONE

Staying in physical contact with your loved one sounds simple, but it becomes more complicated at the later stages of Alzheimer's when bulky hospital equipment and more helping hands come into your life. Here's how Mike and I learned to bridge that gap:

1. Sitting side by side.
Mike and I enjoyed watching television at the end of each day while sitting side by side on the couch. When sitting on the couch became too difficult for Mike, he moved to a chair with firm arm rests.

To keep our side-by-side TV ritual alive, I simply slid my chair next to his. That way we could still lean close to each other or hold hands.

2. Saying hello and goodbye.
Now that other people were in our home caring for Mike, it would have been easy to skip our ritual of hugs and kisses whenever I left or returned to the house. Instead, we continued to kiss and give each other public displays of affection no matter who was present.

3. Staying clean and huggable.
Keeping Mike clean, fresh, well-dressed and well-groomed remained an important part of his day and mine. (Old saying: If you want to be hugged, be huggable.)

4. Reaching out during the day.
There are little opportunities for loving touch, here and there, throughout every day: a pat on the arm, a hand on the shoulder, or simply eye-to-eye contact that only you and your partner know is like a touch. Don't let those slip away!

5. Keeping our marriage bed.
This was a big deal and I devoted the entire previous chapter to how Mike and I continued to sleep close to each other at night. I am convinced it helped both of us sleep better, all the way to the end.

6. Giving massages.
While I did not give Mike full massages like a professional, I did give him relaxing hand and arm massages, especially during the last few weeks of his life when his arms were often tight. Massaging his arms helped him relax and go back to sleep.

In addition, one of the many wonderful services that hospice offered was a massage every other week. Mike, who had never had a massage, was agreeable and it seemed to help both of us unwind. (While he was getting a massage, I escaped to the kitchen for tea.)

INSIGHTS

- I believe that loving touch was definitely therapeutic for Mike throughout his entire Alzheimer's journey, helping him stay connected to me and extending both the length and the quality of his life.

- Massage has a calming effect, not only on the one receiving the massage but the one giving it.

- Despite Alzheimer's, I believe Mike was able to stay connected to me by sight, sound, smell, and definitely by my touch right up to the very last day. Again, loving touch made a real difference!

PART XII

~

Mike and I Say
Goodbye

CHAPTER 52

A LIGHT IN THE DARK

---

*I was learning that the final weeks of
life can be a very spiritual time, if you
just remain open and present with
your loved one.*

ABOUT A WEEK BEFORE MIKE DIED, I was sleeping next to him
in our bedroom. Suddenly I woke to a light I had not seen before. It
seemed to blow in from the window and it settled in the upper left
corner of our room, taking up about a fourth of the ceiling.

I say "blow" for this light flowed like wind, strong at first and
then softer. It was bright enough to wake me, and cause me to wonder where such a light could possibly be coming from. And it was
like no other light I had seen before or have seen since.

At first I thought, "Maybe I didn't close the curtains enough, or
maybe the light was coming over the top of the curtain rod." But
that was not so. I lay quite still, watching the light and expecting it to
disappear, but it didn't. Sometimes it was brighter, and then softer,
but it never faded away.

As I lay there in my twin bed snuggled next to Mike in his hospital bed, the thought struck me at that moment that this light may
have come to take him away. Quietly and carefully I checked to be
sure he was okay. His breathing was still steady and he seemed to be
resting calmly.

I didn't know what to do next. I did not want to wake Mike. I
thought about walking over to the window to look out, but I didn't
want to leave Mike by himself with this mysterious light so present even for a moment. So I simply watched the light flow for what
seemed like a long time.

Sensing no danger, I finally rolled over and simply looked away from the light that would not go away or allow me to sleep. I still felt a little uneasy, but I snuggled closer to Mike and soon fell asleep again.

When I awoke in the morning, the light was gone and Mike was still fine. Clearly, he had had a good night's sleep—much more peaceful than mine.

After that night, however, I noticed that Mike's eyes often went to the same corner of the ceiling where the light had been—a place his eyes had never gone before. That didn't scare me or even surprise me. For now I was learning that the final weeks of life are a spiritual time, if you just remain open and present with your loved one.

There are events in this life that we do not understand; we try to solve their mystery but cannot. Then we have to decide: should we talk about the mystery, let it go, keep it for ourselves or, in my case, include it in a book for all the world to see? Mike's light was one of those.

For a long time I did not talk about the mysterious light and then only told a trusted few. But, as I began to share that experience with others, I discovered that they, too, had very similar stories to tell of the mystery of life and death. And, as I continue to listen and wonder, I discover that I believe a little more and wonder a little less.

CHAPTER 53

LETTING GO

*Now it is time to share what the final
days were like for Mike and me, and
to tell you of our last goodbye.*

IT WAS TIME TO LET MICHAEL GO, BUT COULD I? The sadness
of watching my husband's gradual decline over the final months was
overwhelming at times, bringing me to tears. And yet I was still able
to provide care for him each day, find joy that we were together in
our home, and treasure our afternoon naps and shared bed at night.
I knew in my heart that the time to let Mike go in peace had finally
come, but it was so difficult to accept that soon we would no longer
be together.

I feared the last weeks of Mike's life knowing that people with
Alzheimer's eventually lose their ability to swallow, which means
they cannot eat or drink. I didn't want that to happen to Mike, but
it did. Day by day, he began eating less and less. Then one Saturday
(May 28), when I returned from work, Sabina told me that she had
not been able to get Mike out of bed that day, and he had swallowed
very little food or drink. He went from a swallow or two on Saturday to no swallow at all on Sunday and Monday.

I could see, now, that Mike's death was imminent, perhaps only a
matter of days. It was the beginning of Memorial Day weekend and
I was looking at spending Sunday and Monday on my own. I could
not imagine being all by myself at this critical time, so I called a dear
friend in Seattle to come stay with me. Fortunately, she was there
when I had to make the decision to stop giving Mike food or drink.
That was so hard. All I could do was hold tight to what the hospice

nurse had told me—that those who are nearing the end of life are no longer hungry.

GATHERING OUR LITTLE FAMILY TOGETHER

The next nine days were difficult, but filled with love. Knowing that Mike's days were now numbered, I called our son Patrick who was teaching on the East Coast. I told him I wanted him home with Dad, me and Kathleen—and he came immediately. As we entered this final stage, I felt the need to stay very close to my beloved husband and best friend. One by one I told our dear circle—my sisters, friends, Sabina and Stephanie—that Mike and I no longer needed their help because Patrick and Kathleen were now at the house with me. Our circle of friends and family had been so good to us and had carried us through the months and years of Mike's care. And yet I hoped they would understand that my children and I needed to spend this final time alone with their dad.

Through the last days, Kathleen and Patrick were right there helping with Mike's care and sitting by his side. Often, little Riley and her ever-present doll came too. Mike was not in pain at this point, but we who loved him certainly were.

⭢ FROM MY JOURNAL ⭠
JUNE 1 (WEDNESDAY)

All night Mike's breathing was loud and irregular. I turned him and now slow, shallow breathing—no tension in his body. The only medication last night was one Lorazepam at 9:00 p.m. While I lay next to Mike in the afternoon, he moved his head toward mine and attempted to elevate his arm around me. It felt like he was giving me my last hug.

JUNE 3 (FRIDAY)

This entry may be my last while Mike is still alive. I know I will miss Mike's presence greatly. And yet, more and more each day, I want this to end.

JUNE 4 (SATURDAY)

Mike continues to work so hard to be with us. Please God let him go in peace—give him the love he needs to know it is okay to go. This is so hard.

JUNE 5 (SUNDAY)

This morning I said to Mike, "Soon you will be on a new adventure. You will know one of the great mysteries of life." (Then talked about family and friends who had died.)

SAYING GOODBYE

I had heard along the way that it is sometimes necessary for those who love someone who is dying to let them go. I did not know what "letting go" was all about, but now I was learning. As the days without food or water wore on, I did all that I could to let Mike know that, when he was ready, I, too, was prepared to let him go.

Now when I sat next to him at the side of the bed or lay near his side for our little talks, I gently let him hear that it was okay for him to die. I assured him that he was a good father and had been a good provider, that we would be okay when he needed to depart, that I loved him so much, that we had done a good job working together, that we were still here together in our home, and that Patrick and Kathleen were here too.

Throughout the last seven days of Mike's life, Patrick, Kathleen, and I spent most of our waking hours in the room with him. We often lay on the bed next to him or sat near his side, now just our little family. Stories were told of times gone by, and we always assumed Mike was listening to every word.

Patrick often talked aloud about the old days and the good times with his dad, while Kathleen preferred alone time at his bedside. When we were together in the room we talked easily and naturally, just as we had for so many years, about the day, the weather, good memories, what Riley had done and of the current moment. And, of course, there were times when one or the other of us became overwhelmed with emotion and had to step out of the room.

Then, on the ninth day of no food or drink, I lay next to Mike after our afternoon nap together, and we looked into each other's eyes. I could tell Mike was listening closely as we had this one last talk and I said something just a little different:

> "This is really hard now, Mike.
> We have done everything we can.
> We have had a wonderful life together.
> It is now time for you to go.
> I will miss you, but know that I will join you someday soon.
> This Alzheimer's has been hard, but we did it right.
> You have done such a good job and now your work is done."

There was one long look, eye to eye, a kiss, and then his gaze once again moved up to the corner of the ceiling. I assured him I would soon be back and stepped out of the room. I checked on him one more time about 20 minutes later, gave him one last kiss and one more "I love you."

Mike died at 5:50 p.m., June 6, 2011, in the bedroom of our home right where he wanted to be. He had hoped beyond hope that this dread disease would not make him leave his home or rob him of his family and wife, and it had not. Our children were with us every step of the way and Mike and I were still in love, perhaps even more at that moment than ever before. The disease had not pulled us apart as we had feared, but had brought us a new respect for each other and a love that just grew deeper day by day.

Rev. Dennis Tierney delivered a beautiful eulogy for Michael— one that captures his spirit and placed a fitting end on our long journey with Alzheimer's. I've included his eulogy in part for you in the next chapter.

- Many say that Alzheimer's patients are not aware during the last couple years of their illness, and especially at the very end, but that was not my experience with Mike. We never gave up consciously connecting with each other, even when he was at his most impaired.

- One of the greatest gifts our friend from Seattle provided was her memory of what happened that Memorial Day weekend. She reminded me that every time I turned Mike or settled him he would pucker up and give me silent kisses. Not just this, but many other subtle efforts by Mike convinced me that he still knew me and loved me at the very end.

- Despite all the difficulties of the final year, Mike continued to share priceless moments with his family. Even as his abilities went into severe decline, his continued presence provided love in our family right up to the day he died.

- Some people die when their loved one steps out of the room for just a moment, and that was the case with Mike and me. I kissed him and stepped away for just a short time, and that's when he let go and died. Why this happens is unknown. Deborah Sigrist, in her book *Journey's End*, says some want to spare certain loved ones from the dying moment. Perhaps that's what Mike intended. Perhaps he was giving me one last gift.

CHAPTER 54

FOREVER REMEMBERED

*To live in the hearts we leave
behind is not to die.*
—Thomas Campbell

IT WAS JULY 23RD, a balmy summer's day on Bainbridge Island, when we all gathered at St. Barnabas Church for Mike's memorial.

The church was full. Many faces were familiar to me; others were unknown, but all had arrived that day with love in their hearts for my courageous husband. There was sadness, of course, but also joy for a life well-led—and respect, too, for a battle well-fought.

Our dear minister, the Rev. Dennis Tierney, gave the perfect eulogy; I knew Mike would have been proud of the words Dennis chose. Here is the excerpt I especially want to share with you.

~

LOVE NEVER ENDS
(MIKE'S EULOGY BY REV. DENNIS TIERNEY)

Mike Peel was a courageous man. That courage served him well in his illness. When faced with a terrible diagnosis he simply said, "Let's get on with it." There was no pity party for him. He ran to joy all the days of his life…

Mike loved his wife and family deeply. He adored his granddaughter Riley and delighted in her presence. His love was the kind Saint Paul talks about. It was patient and kind, it bore all things and endured all things. Mike Peel experienced the unkindest of diseases and yet never lost his ability to love and show love.

(continued next page)

As Rosalys shared with me, in the end, when all of Mike's abilities were diminished or gone, Mike could still show his love. When all other forms of communication had been taken, Mike could still raise an eyebrow and show love. He could still make the shape of a kiss with his lips and send it to those he loved. And when asked, "Where is your wedding ring?"— that sign of marital love and commitment —Mike could still move his ring finger.

Yes, life may end, but love never ends. For the last ten years of his life, Mike's physical world slipped away. But his love endured; it remained as bright and powerful as it had always been. True love never ends.

But what of us? Mike is now whole and at peace; fully embraced in the love of God. It is for us, the living, to consider how we might best remember this wonderful man. One thing we can do is to see the world with all its difficulties squarely and clearly but go on loving it anyway. There we have it: love as he did, run to joy as he did, and just get on with it as he did.

~

MIKE'S LEGACY CONTINUES

Yes, Mike died at the end of his journey, just as we all die some day, it's part of our humanity. But I know Mike would say that each of us should die only once instead of dying every day by letting Alzheimer's steal the joy and peace of mind from whatever precious time we are given.

Through ten years, Mike and I refused to dwell on dying and focused instead on living. We knew that new breakthroughs in Alzheimer's treatment were possibly right around the corner. But even if Mike did not live long enough to benefit from those breakthroughs, we hoped to still come to the end of his life together, still in our home and still in love. We did, and now my highest hope is that you and your loved one will achieve your highest hopes too.

This, then, is the most enduring part of Mike's legacy: Alzheimer's may be a formidable opponent, but let the example of Mike's life remind you that Alzheimer's can never extinguish our love. It cannot suppress our faith. It cannot diminish our courage or our sense of humor. It cannot end our friendship or our compassion. It cannot vanquish our spirit—and it cannot steal eternal life.

PART XIII

~

Hope for the Future

CHAPTER 55

HAVE FAITH

*We are winning the war on
Alzheimer's — it's happening —
and you and your loved one are on
the front lines of this emerging story.*

AS I WAS FINISHING THIS BOOK, the Alzheimer's Association launched an inspiring national ad campaign. Below is an excerpt from that campaign. I hope this message speaks directly to you and your loved one at this point in your journey.

WHEN WE REACH THE FIRST SURVIVOR

"The first person to survive Alzheimer's disease
is out there now.
That person is going to hold on
to everything the disease steals away...
Every single piece of them
is going to make it through.
And the Alzheimer's Association
is going to make it happen
by funding research, advancing public
policy, and spurring scientific breakthroughs.
And by providing local support for
those living with the disease and their caregivers.
Alzheimer's has devastated millions of lives,
but that's all going to change
when we reach the first survivor."

— *The Alzheimer's Association*

MY HOPE FOR YOU

The average stone-age human lived to be just 18 years old. But down through the centuries, we've dramatically increased the length and quality of human life—and that long-running success story is still unfolding.

Today, the average American can look forward to living well into their seventies, eighties or longer. Thanks to continuous medical advancements we now give new hearts, eyes and limbs to the sick or injured. Together we have virtually wiped out scarlet fever, small-pox, polio and a dozen other fearsome illnesses—and we are now gaining ground on cancer and Alzheimer's too.

We have learned from long experience that the best way to defeat a bully like Alzheimer's is to come together and gang up on the disease. Remember always that you and your loved one are not alone. Today, thousands of Alzheimer's researchers, doctors, nurses, care-givers, long-term care facilities and hospice workers are fighting this disease on several fronts; and we are combining the best of what we're learning to improve care for everyone—and to find a cure.

One of the most important fronts, of course, is the home front. *Mike & Me* is one of several new books to chronicle the changing face of home care among Alzheimer's couples. Together, we are learning how the astonishing power of love, patience, compassion and stay-at-home care can help Alzheimer's patients defy the usual statistics and live a longer, fuller life.

It's my great hope that within these pages you have found fresh information to bring you and your loved one peace of mind and heart, along with some new and important tips. But, above all else, I pray that *Mike & Me* will bring you renewed hope and courage for the journey ahead.

CHAPTER 56

WE ARE ALL IN THIS
FIGHT TOGETHER

*It is my very great hope that each of
us in our own way will help create
a wider circle of compassion and
support for all who have Alzheimer's.*

THE NUMBER OF PEOPLE LIVING WITH ALZHEIMER'S IS GROW-
ING. As I write this chapter, one in every ten people over age 65
across the nation is coping with the disease. In fact, if everyone
with Alzheimer's started wearing a yellow ribbon on their arm, you
would suddenly see yellow ribbons everywhere you go. And yet it is
not unusual for Alzheimer's couples to feel overlooked and alone in
our culture. Why is that?

Part of the reason is that many goodhearted people literally don't
know how to react when they notice a person with Alzheimer's or
dementia in their midst. In the final years of the disease, I could see
that some people immediately felt uncomfortable when Mike and
I would enter a public place. They didn't want to stare, or say the
wrong thing, or seem impolite, so they would simply pretend that
they didn't notice us.

Throughout this book I have spoken with gratitude about our
circle of close friends and family who helped Mike and me as the
disease progressed. Now I want to tell you how each of us in our
own way can help create a wider circle of compassion and support
for all who have Alzheimer's. It's easier than you might imagine. You
won't have to give a lot of time, effort or money to make a difference
for people with Alzheimer's; you just have to be willing to give a

welcoming smile, a listening ear, or a helpful hand now and then. Here's a little story that will show you what I mean:

HOW LITTLE THINGS CAN MAKE A BIG DIFFERENCE

Recently, while driving to Montana, I pulled in at a rest stop. While sitting at one of the picnic tables, I watched people come and go and noticed one couple in particular. It was easy to see that the husband had Alzheimer's or dementia. I noticed how his wife patiently gave him instructions before sending him into the men's room by himself—and then she went off to the lady's room.

A few moments later, however, the husband wandered out of the restroom, turned right, and began walking toward the highway. Alarmed, I saw that this was a moment when I could give a helping hand to a stranger. Strolling toward him, I greeted the confused gentleman and commented on the beautiful day. He seemed content to stop and talk with a lady who was willing to carry the conversation, so I continued on.

"I am headed to Montana," I told him cheerfully, "are you going to Seattle?" It seemed that he was, so I talked a little about where I lived. Soon his wife was by our side and pleased to see a caring person talking with her husband.

We had a brief conversation and she told me that her husband had Alzheimer's and it had gotten so hard. I was careful how I spoke, always looking to include her husband in the conversation, just as I had always done with Mike. It was easy to smile, make eye contact and include him. I told him that my husband, too, had sometimes forgotten which way to go, but we still had loved taking trips together.

Before leaving, the wife took my hand and said how grateful she was that I had reached out to help her husband. I wanted her to know that I understood and reminded her that she was not alone. I watched as they walked away, content and happy, side by side. For a moment I was a little sad that I no longer had Mike to travel the road with me. But it was a good feeling to know that I had been able to give two strangers—a fellow Alzheimer's couple—a helping hand. And then I thought of all those who had done the same for Mike and me through the years.

You can see how easy it was for me to stop, smile and reach out to my fellow travelers in a way that made a difference in their day. I like to think that if I had not stopped my new friend from wandering toward the highway, someone else would have noticed and stepped in. What I am uncertain about is whether or not someone else would have spoken to him as an equal. My hope is that this book will help all of us remember that those who are coping with Alzheimer's are still very much with us and far more aware than most of us might think.

LET'S ALL REACH OUT

As our nation becomes more aware of the six million Americans with Alzheimer's, it's my great hope that all of us will reach out with kindness and compassion whenever we see an Alzheimer's couple who could use a smile or a helping hand. What a difference it would make if everyone was willing to open a door for a caregiver, or smile at an Alzheimer's couple, or take a moment to speak to them on the train, or in the museum, or at a rest stop.

Finally, here is one especially important suggestion about reaching out to people with Alzheimer's. As the disease progressed, Mike naturally had more and more difficulty participating in a conversation, especially with people he had just met. Often he would simply let me do the talking for both of us. The reaction from whomever we were speaking with was almost always the same: Since Mike wasn't actively engaged in the conversation, they quit making eye contact with him, and carried on the conversation solely with me. This made Mike feel as if he was no longer included or valuable.

Please don't fall into the trap of talking to the caregiver without acknowledging the person with Alzheimer's. Continue to smile and make eye contact with them, even though they may not seem like they are tracking the conversation. The truth is, a person with Alzheimer's usually knows and feels much more than people give them credit for. Your kind and compassionate acknowledgment of their presence in your conversation can mean the world to them.

As Mother Teresa reminds us, "We shall never know all the good a simple smile and a caring word can do."

―――――――――――――― **INSIGHTS** ――――――――――――――

- Being Mike's caregiver was never easy, but it brought me so many unforeseen gifts and helped me see things differently. Now, for example, whenever I see people in wheelchairs and those who care for them, I know neither has an easy job. If I can stop in my day to open a door or give them a helping hand, then I am there!

- No couple can go it alone with Alzheimer's. We all need caring friends and family to keep us on our feet, lend a helping hand, or pick us up when we are down. Thank you, one and all, you know who you are.

CHAPTER 57

THE MAILBOX AT THE
TOP OF THE HILL

As time passed, that familiar walk up
our driveway took on new meaning
for Mike and me.

MIKE LOVED TO READ THE NEWSPAPER from cover to cover.
When he was still working, he would always stop to pick up the
morning paper as he drove out the driveway on his way to the ferry.
A cup of coffee, a ferry ride, and his friend the newspaper were the
perfect start for the day.

After he retired, he enjoyed the short daily walk up our driveway
to get the newspaper and the mail. After he was diagnosed with Alzheimer's, the walk to the mailbox became an important ritual—a
way to be independent, a sign of everyday normality. It was also an
opportunity to chat with whoever might be about—the postal person, our ninety-year-old neighbor, the folks working in the neighborhood, and often Merlin—the Golden Retriever—who lived
next door and was the recipient of many warm and friendly pats
and back scratches from Mike.

As Alzheimer's progressed, that familiar walk up the driveway
became a challenge. Still, Mike liked the walk, and I enjoyed watching him journey up the driveway on his own for as long as possible.
At first he walked up the slope with a bounce in his step, sometimes
with a little run, then more slowly as I watched out the window to
be sure he turned in the right direction to come back to the house.

As time went on, he started having trouble remembering which
box was ours and would frequently return with the neighbor's

newspaper or mail. This was such an important job of his—getting the newspaper in the morning and the mail in the afternoon. But how could he continue his job if he could no longer recognize our mailbox?

One day, while feeling inspired, I wrapped bright yellow tape around our mailbox and the newspaper box. I wondered, would Mike remember the yellow tape was our box? I'm not sure if it helped, but the bright yellow tape did make Mike, me and the neighbors all smile.

In fact our teenage neighbor, Signe, told me that the morning mailbox ritual was how the neighbors knew how Mike was doing.

Time marched on: At first Mike walked to the mailbox by himself. Then we walked together. Next, our granddaughter joined us, first as a baby in the stroller, and later as a toddler with one hand on grandpa's wheelchair.

Today, I walk to the yellow-taped mailbox with two giggling grandchildren. Mike is no longer with us, but he is.

ACKNOWLEDGMENTS

My SINCERE THANKS to all who made "Mike & Me" possible, including and especially the following:

To our courageous children Patrick and Kathleen, this story would not have had the same ending, were it not for your tireless love, understanding and support from the very beginning to the very end. And to our son-in-law Sam Hadley who did all that he could for us and was the support team for Kathleen and little Riley too.

To my sisters: Patty Meritt who repeatedly saved the day by traveling from Alaska and staying long weekends with Mike so I could continue to teach and have a night away; and Gerrie Harper who was always just a phone call away.

To our kind and compassionate caregivers Stephanie Davenport and Sabina Price who knew how to listen and support, and still carry on through even the most difficult days. We could not have continued on without your gentle ways.

To our good friends Stan & Audrey Van Voorhis, and Arthur & Wendy Davenport, you were always right there when we needed your love and support the most. And to our ever-vigilant neighbors Gary & Linda Quitslund and Kirt Alquist, I knew you were standing by for Mike and me, day or night.

To our California team who just kept coming with more love, laughter and listening ears, thank you: Margaret & Mike Gaines, Marilyn Tobin, Claudia Kreis, Shirley Resich, and sister Roberta Halverson.

To our cousins who each found a way to help in their own special way: Andy Meritt, Paul Meritt, Mattie Davies & brother-in-law Bob Meritt, the Harper clan, Tim & Cherie Graves, John & Joreen Graves.

To Rev. Dennis Tierney and our faith community at St Barnabas. You gave us spiritual help at Sunday morning services as well as in the quiet of our home. You will never know what a difference your prayers and kindness made to Mike and me.

To Dr. Jung who guided every stage of our journey for ten years, constantly showing us what was possible and alerting us to what lie ahead. And to all the unsung heroes on our hospice team, including Betty our hospice aide. You brought us courage, comfort and compassion through the final days.

To Bernie Fischer and Amy Dapice, thank you for carrying the torch for us part of the way, and for cheering us on to the end. Your high intention made a difference.

To our gifted art director and tenacious copy editor Toby and Luana Cowan of Performance Design Group. Your creativity and friendship filled me with confidence and joy, and made every page look and read just right.

And to Dan Zadra, my extraordinary editor, publisher and kindred spirit. It was no coincidence that a chance meeting brought you into my life as I fumbled at making this dream come true. Thank you, Dan, for being such a good listener, for your expert guidance in helping me write this story with clarity and integrity, and for giving time and energy beyond my wildest expectations. You were with me every step of the way. I thank you for your kindness, vision, and tenacity. Most of all I thank you for believing in a project from the very first day that will, hopefully, guide and inspire many couples who are now on their own Alzheimer's journey.

MORE PRAISE FOR *MIKE & ME*

"As a hospice nurse I was touched by this couple's endless devotion and commitment to each other. This book is a vital guide for couples confronting the challenges of Alzheimer's, as well as professionals working with the families."
— **Barbara Konikow, R.N.**, Hospice Nurse

"A priceless guide for Alzheimer's couples, with fresh insights from the loving spouse's point of view. It's a book about true love, integrity, courage and being there for one another, even when there are no other words to say. This is one book we all may turn to at some point in our lives!"
— **Jennifer C. Hurwitz**, Legacies of Cincinnati Cancer Support Community

"Rich with insight, validation, tools, and anecdotes that deepen our ability to support each other in all the ways dementia touches our lives. It is recommended not only for partners of those with dementia, but also family and clinical professionals working to keep people with memory loss and their caregivers supported in the community."
— **Brian Osborn**, Manager of PACE Operations, Providence ElderPlace

"This book is a wise and heartfelt guide for couples and families facing Alzheimer's. The author shows couples how to avoid becoming victims of the disease. Through love and perseverance, she shows us instead how to take the helm and navigate the storms with grace and dignity."
— **R. Louise Smyth, M.D.**

"A loving guide for spouses, family members and friends dealing with Alzheimer's (but really any progressive or terminal illness). The author's insights are spot-on and she doesn't hesitate to admit

where she made mistakes along the way, in order to help her readers avoid them."
—**Amy Reichbach**

"What a gift to couples dealing with Alzheimer's! In her candid stories and touching journal entries, Rosalys Peel shows how one couple learned to confront the travails of Alzheimer's together—and managed to stay deeply in love throughout the entire journey."
— **Karen Carson**, Educator/Support Group Facilitator

"I treasure this book. To see great negotiation, read the gentle chapter on driving privileges. To share true joy, read the chapter on daughter Kathleen's wedding. To find good sound advice, read any chapter. You will find subtle grace, determination and love that will help you along your trail, wherever it may lead."
— **Mike Henderson**

"*Mike & Me* is a must-have for any couple touched by Alzheimer's. Wise and compassionate with a powerful thread of common sense, the book guides us fearlessly through the ups and downs, pitfalls and breakthroughs of this generation's most misunderstood disease."
— **Tom Horton**, former CEO, HL2

"*Mike & Me* is an inspiring how-to guide for couples dealing with the challenges of Alzheimer's at home. It's the story of two people who refused to take the typical path and set out instead on a courageous Alzheimer's journey of their own."
— **Anne Zadra**, Author, *The House at the Bottom of the Hill*

"Any couple experiencing the challenges of Alzheimer's can turn confidently to this book. They will find themselves picking it up over and over throughout the journey for inspiration, encouragement and very good advice."
— **Brian Lee**, Silver Valley Writers

ABOUT THE AUTHOR

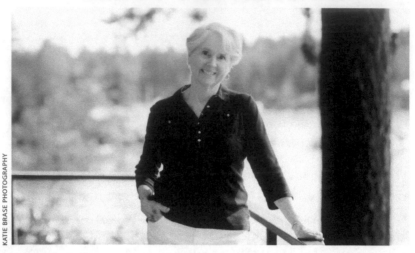

ROSALYS PEEL is a Registered Nurse, a Lamaze-certified childbirth educator, and a Gottman-certified couples' relationship facilitator. For over 30 years she has been a respected voice in the childbirth education movement. She currently teaches classes at Swedish Medical Center in Seattle and has been a featured guest on NPR and *The Today Show*.

When her husband Mike was stricken with Alzheimer's, Rosalys searched the bookshelves for a "couple's guide" that would show them how to deal with Mike's illness together at home. Unable to find that book, she came back after her husband's death from Alzheimer's to write it herself.

Mike & Me draws on ten years of her journal notes along with her unique background in birth and family education.

Rosalys lives on Bainbridge Island, Washington, near her children and grandchildren, just a brief ferry ride from Seattle. She remains a tireless teacher, writer, speaker, and a caring advocate for Alzheimer's couples.

DAN ZADRA is the Creative Director of Zadra Publishing, and the founder and former creative director of Compendium Publishing in Seattle. He has edited, authored or co-authored dozens of award-winning books over the past 30 years, including six consecutive bestsellers. He currently lives and writes in Wallace, Idaho, where he collaborated with Rosalys Peel on *Mike & Me* for Alzheimer's couples.

SHARE YOUR THOUGHTS

With the Author:
Your thoughts will be forwarded immediately to
Rosalys Peel when you send them to:
DearRosalys@ZadraCreative.com

With Zadra Publishing:
Submit your review of Mike&Me in writing to:
Publisher@ZadraCreative.com

For more resources for Alzheimer's couples
and caregivers, visit:
www.MikeandMeBook.com

An imprint of Zadra Creative, LLC
513½ Bank St.
Suite A
Wallace, Idaho 83873

CPSIA information can be obtained
at www.ICGtesting.com
Printed in the USA
LVHW050828270219
608902LV00007B/147